EAI/Springer Innovations in Communication and Computing

Series editor
Imrich Chlamtac, European Alliance for Innovation, Gent, Belgium

Editor's Note

The impact of information technologies is creating a new world yet not fully understood. The extent and speed of economic, life style and social changes already perceived in everyday life is hard to estimate without understanding the technological driving forces behind it. This series presents contributed volumes featuring the latest research and development in the various information engineering technologies that play a key role in this process.

The range of topics, focusing primarily on communications and computing engineering include, but are not limited to, wireless networks; mobile communication; design and learning; gaming; interaction; e-health and pervasive healthcare; energy management; smart grids; internet of things; cognitive radio networks; computation; cloud computing; ubiquitous connectivity, and in mode general smart living, smart cities, Internet of Things and more. The series publishes a combination of expanded papers selected from hosted and sponsored European Alliance for Innovation (EAI) conferences that present cutting edge, global research as well as provide new perspectives on traditional related engineering fields. This content, complemented with open calls for contribution of book titles and individual chapters, together maintain Springer's and EAI's high standards of academic excellence. The audience for the books consists of researchers, industry professionals, advanced level students as well as practitioners in related fields of activity include information and communication specialists, security experts, economists, urban planners, doctors, and in general representatives in all those walks of life affected ad contributing to the information revolution.

About EAI

EAI is a grassroots member organization initiated through cooperation between businesses, public, private and government organizations to address the global challenges of Europe's future competitiveness and link the European Research community with its counterparts around the globe. EAI reaches out to hundreds of thousands of individual subscribers on all continents and collaborates with an institutional member base including Fortune 500 companies, government organizations, and educational institutions, provide a free research and innovation platform.

Through its open free membership model EAI promotes a new research and innovation culture based on collaboration, connectivity and recognition of excellence by community.

More information about this series at http://www.springer.com/series/15427

Pedro R. M. Inácio • Ana Duarte • Paulo Fazendeiro
Nuno Pombo
Editors

5th EAI International Conference on IoT Technologies for HealthCare

Springer

EAI
RESEARCH MEETS INNOVATION

Editors
Pedro R. M. Inácio
Instituto de Telecomunicações
Universidade da Beira Interior
Covilhã, Portugal

Ana Duarte
Department of Health Sciences
Universidade da Beira Interior
Covilhã, Portugal

Paulo Fazendeiro
Instituto de Telecomunicações
Universidade da Beira Interior
Covilhã, Portugal

Nuno Pombo
Instituto de Telecomunicações
Universidade da Beira Interior
Covilhã, Portugal

ISSN 2522-8595 ISSN 2522-8609 (electronic)
EAI/Springer Innovations in Communication and Computing
ISBN 978-3-030-30334-1 ISBN 978-3-030-30335-8 (eBook)
https://doi.org/10.1007/978-3-030-30335-8

This Springer imprint is published by the registered company Springer Nature Switzerland AG.
The registered company address is: Gewerbestrasse 11, 6330 Cham, Switzerland

Preface

The Internet of Things, a paradigm leveraging a set of existing and emerging technologies, notions, and services, can provide many solutions to delivery of electronic healthcare, patient care, and medical data management. The proceedings of the fifth edition of the European Alliance for Innovation (EAI) International Conference on Internet of Things Technologies for Healthcare (HealthyIoT 2018) are a representative snapshot of the ongoing research efforts being made to achieve these goals.

The technical program of HealthyIoT 2018 consisted of two keynote speeches (*IoT Sensors in the Framework of Aging in Place* and *Pervasive Electrocardiography* delivered, respectively, by the researchers Bart Vanrumste and Hugo Silva) and 10 papers encompassing basic and applied research in themes as diverse as the study of materials for mobile off-the-person ECG, the use of intelligent phonocardiography for screening pediatric heart disease, the monitoring of respiratory rate for early detection of diseases, the sleep detection with wearable devices, the remote rehabilitation via exergaming, the study of EMG sensors for a bionic hand, the future expectations on telemonitoring devices and systems, the security solutions for e-health information systems, and the development of ontologies to manage the huge amounts of heterogeneous medical devices and data.

There are sets of different actors that have contributed to the success of this meeting. First of all, we are in debt to the authors who generously have submitted and shared their most recent research endeavors. We also commend the hard work of the members of the Technical Program Committee for being part of the peer-review process of technical papers thus ensuring a high-quality technical program. It was also a great pleasure to work with the excellent organizing committee team for their hard work in organizing and supporting the conference. Last, but not least, we also appreciate the constant support and guidance from the steering chair, Imrich Chlamtac, and from the always-present Conference Managers.

As a final remark, we sincerely believe that HealthyIoT has succeeded in bringing together technology experts, researchers, industry and international authorities that are nowadays contributing towards the design, development and deployment of healthcare solutions based on IoT technologies, standards, and procedures.

Covilhã, Portugal Pedro R. M. Inácio
Covilhã, Portugal Ana Duarte
Covilhã, Portugal Paulo Fazendeiro
Covilhã, Portugal Nuno Pombo

Conference Organization

Steering Committee

Chair

Imrich Chlamtac	Bruno Kessler Professor, University of Trento, Italy

General Co-Chairs

Pedro R. M. Inácio	Universidade da Beira Interior
Ana Paula Duarte	Universidade da Beira Interior
Paulo Fazendeiro	Universidade da Beira Interior
Miguel Castelo Branco	Universidade da Beira Interior
Manuel Lemos	Universidade da Beira Interior

Technical Program Committee Chair

Nuno Pombo	Universidade da Beira Interior

Publications Chair

Paulo Fazendeiro	Universidade da Beira Interior

Publicity and Social Media Chair

Diogo Fernandes	Booking.com

Workshop Chair

Pedro Dinis Gaspar	Universidade da Beira Interior

Web Chair

Bernardo Sequeiros	Universidade da Beira Interior

Conference Manager

Marek Kaleta	EAI
Kristina Lappyova	EAI

Technical Program Committee

Paula Prata	Universidade da Beira Interior, Portugal
Pedro Araújo	Universidade da Beira Interior, Portugal
Luisa Jorge	Instituto Politécnico de Bragança, Portugal
Ivan Chorbev	Ss. Cyril and Methodius University, FYR of Macedonia
Eftim Zdravevski	Ss. Cyril and Methodius University, FYR of Macedonia
Vladimir Trajkovik	Ss. Cyril and Methodius University, FYR of Macedonia
Bruno Silva	Universidade Europeia, Portugal
Emmanuel Conchon	XLIM – University of Limoges, France.
Zdenka Babic	University of Banja Luka, Bosnia and Herzegovina
Johanna Virkki	Tampere University of Technology, Finland
Sari Merilampi	Satakunta University of Applied Sciences, Finland
Peter Pocta	University of Zilina, Slovakia
Aleksandar Jevremovic	Singidunum University, Serbia
Marko Sarac	Singidunum University, Serbia
Giannis Gialelis	University of Patras, Greece
Francisco Florez Revuelta	University of Alicante, Spain
Magdalena Punceva	University of Applied Sciences and Arts Western Switzerland
Victor Hugo Albuquerque	University of Fortaleza, Brazil
Imen Megdiche	Institut de Recherche en Informatique de Toulouse, France
Ennio Gambi	Università Politecnica delle Marche, Italy
Stein Kristiansen	University of Oslo, Norway

Contents

Part I
Devices and Materials

Study of Mechanomyographic Alternatives to EMG Sensors for a Low-Cost Open Source Bionic Hand

Joana Marques, Sara Ramos, Milton P. Macedo, and Hugo Plácido da Silva

1 Introduction

Owing to the huge evolution in the sensor and microprocessor technologies, as well as in 3D (Three-Dimensional) printing, the development of prosthesis has undergone a great transformation. Particularly for the hand, the myoelectric solution is still the choice of the majority of amputees, although limited by the prohibitive price of bionic hands. Differences are in the versatility of each solution, because in the myoelectric case the hand is opened and closed being able to grasp objects. In opposition, bionic hands are capable of executing individual motions of the fingers, subsequently having a higher functionality approaching the human hand. There is a plethora of commercial hands with a wide range of costs; two of them are shown in Fig. 1. Its cost greatly varies from 5 to 50 k euros, for Open Bionics and Michelangelo hands.

The aim of this work is to study the effectiveness of low-cost sensors for the replacement of EMG (ElectroMyography) sensors commonly used for upper-limb prosthesis. Any movement/gesture executed by a human hand is triggered by command signals sent by the brain, and it implies the ability of nervous cells

J. Marques · S. Ramos
Instituto Politécnico de Coimbra, ISEC, DFM, Rua Pedro Nunes, Quinta da Nora, Coimbra, Portugal

M. P. Macedo (✉)
Instituto Politécnico de Coimbra, ISEC, DFM, Rua Pedro Nunes, Quinta da Nora, Coimbra, Portugal

LIBPhys, Department of Physics, University of Coimbra, Rua Larga, Coimbra, Portugal
e-mail: mpmacedo@isec.pt

H. P. da Silva
IT - Instituto de Telecomunicações, Lisbon, Portugal

P. R. M. Inácio et al. (eds.), *5th EAI International Conference on IoT Technologies for HealthCare*, EAI/Springer Innovations in Communication and Computing,
https://doi.org/10.1007/978-3-030-30335-8_1

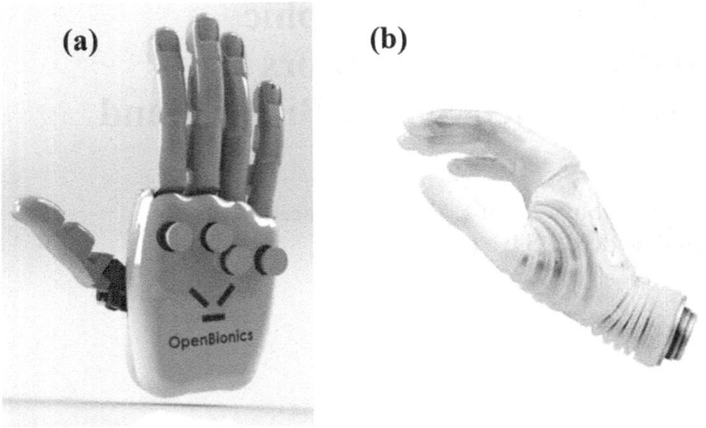

Fig. 1 Examples of commercial hands. Open Bionics (**a**) and Michelangelo (**b**)

to transmit electrical signals. In the typical approach, EMG sensors acquire these myoelectric signals through electrodes placed in appropriate locations, taking into consideration the muscles involved in each movement.

Surface-mounted electrodes are preferably used in case muscles provide signals with enough intensity to be detected. These electrodes, placed on the skin surface, capture the aggregated activity within the area of detection. Three electrodes are used with their locations being chosen depending on the muscles activated in a certain gesture. One of the electrodes is the ground electrode, typically placed in a bone region (electrical neutral) and the other two are active electrodes that collect a signal whose amplitude is proportional to the electrical activity differential between them, and also to the electrode area.

In spite of the typical approach of using EMG signals, there are some drawbacks that have led to the attempts of extracting other type of information, namely to predict muscle forces from EMG signals using the wavelet transform [1]. One of those drawbacks is the often degradation of EMG signals due to electromagnetic interference which implies a large processing time for features extraction [2].

In contrast, the mechanical change of the muscles can be measured by a method with sensitivity to the position/motion of a small area in surface of the muscle, and is typically known as MMG (MechanoMyography). The possibility of acquiring a mechanical deformation map seems potentially interesting as the shape of the muscles changes when different sets of fingers are moved. It has already been implemented using FSR (Force Sensitive Resistor) [2]. Also the application of load cells is described in literature [3].

Another obvious choice to detect mechanical changes is light instrumentation. Amongst the vast offer in these types of sensors, affordable options are available that integrate, in a single package, a light source and detector that could be easily linked to a biosignals acquisition hardware platform.

In this paper we describe and present the results of the application of two MMG sensors and their comparison with EMG signals. Those MMG sensors, an FSR and an IR (InfraRed) reflectance sensor, have shown successful results in gesture recognition and a high SNR (Signal-to-Noise Ratio) in spite of a lower ability to detect different gestures.

2 Materials and Methods

2.1 Sensors

As already mentioned, the reference signal in the scope of this work is the EMG signal. A BITalino EMG sensor was used, which is capable of measuring signals with maximum amplitude of ±1.65 mV and frequencies in the range of 10–400 Hz. A summary of the main specifications can be found in Table 1.

One option for obtaining MMG signal is to use a force sensor in order to react to changes in the muscle volumes, for which an FSR 400 sensor (Interlink Electronics, USA) was selected. It is capable of sensing forces from 0.1 to 10 N (Newton) and it has a circular form factor with 7.62 mm in diameter. A summary of the main specifications can be found in Table 1. The force sensitivity is dependent on the electronic circuit used to achieve the force-to-voltage conversion, which can be realized using a voltage divider followed by an op-amp.

Finally, a third sensor was used in this study to extract features related with the variations in light reflected at the skin surface, as a result of the changes in muscle volume due to the contraction. For the acquisition of this data, a QTR-1A reflectance sensor (Pololu Corporation, USA) was used. It includes an IR LED (InfraRed Light Emitting Diode) and a phototransistor, and the output varies proportionally to the amount of light reflected on a surface. As the light intensity increases (i.e., greater reflection occurs), the lower is the output voltage. It is able to measure a maximum distance of 6 mm, with an optimal sensing distance of 3 mm.

Table 1 Main specifications of each sensor

EMG module specifications	
Gain	1000
Range	±1.65 mV
Bandwidth	10–400 Hz
FSR 400 specifications	
Force sensitivity range	0.1–10.0 N
Force repeatability	±2%
Number of actuations (life time)	Ten million
QTR-1A reflectance sensor specifications	
Optimal sensing distance	3 mm
Maximum sensing distance	6 mm

2.2 Data Acquisition

For this study each sensor was placed individually and acquisitions were carried out using similar timing parameters. The sampling data from four healthy subjects (two men, two women) is summarized in Table 2, from which it is possible to observe that, in each acquisition, the same gesture is made three times. Each gesture lasts for approximately 3 s with similar rest time between them. It is also important to explain that for FSR and IR sensors the acquisition of data from other gestures besides open and close would require the design of a new holder for its fixation and placement that can adapt two or more sensor units.

The acquisition of the signals from each sensor is performed through the hardware platform BITalino Plugged[1]; its OpenSignals software enables real-time data acquisition and recording in a CSV (Comma-Separated Values) format. These data is subsequently used in Matlab[2] (MathWorks, Inc.) for data processing and analysis.

An extremely important issue for the acquisition of signals from any of these three sensors, with a fair signal-to-noise ratio and appropriate sensitivity, is a correct placement of the sensors. Photos of the placement of each of the three sensors are shown in Fig. 2.

From preliminary signal acquisition different strategies were implemented for each sensor, taking into account their sensing parameters. EMG signals were acquired using three pre-gelled electrodes, whose correct placements were chosen taking into consideration the data available in literature [4].

In the case of FSR signals, initially two different positions were tested for open and close gestures, but no features could be extracted. Because of its operation, the IR (reflectance) sensor has different requirements for its placement. It was found that the placement in the two different positions shown in Fig. 2 is suitable to detect open and close gestures.

Table 2 Summary of sampling data

Sensor	Gesture	#Acquisitions	#Muscle activations
EMG	Open	18	54
	Close	24	72
	Point	13	39
FSR	Open	18	42
	Close	32	96
IR	Open	16	48
	Close	20	60

[1]http://bitalino.com/datasheets/BITalino_Plugged_Datasheet.pdf.

[2]https://www.mathworks.com/products/matlab.html.

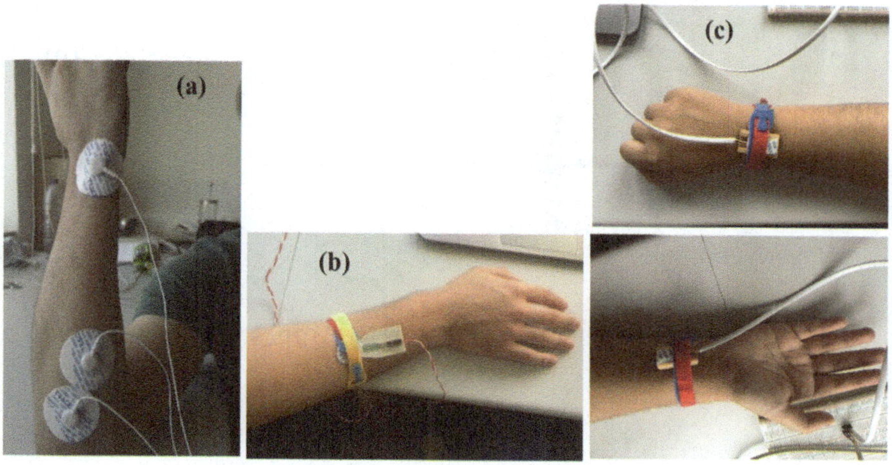

Fig. 2 Photos of the sensors placement. Three EMG pre-gelled electrodes (**a**), FSR sensor with velcro strap for fixation (**b**), and IR sensor mounted inside a 3D printed fixation support and velcro strap for fixation (**c**)

2.3 Data Processing

For FSR and IR sensors, raw data was used in spite of a variable baseline that eventually could be corrected through the use of the derivative of these signals. The EMG sensor is used in a bipolar differential front-end for a higher signal-to-noise ratio. Firstly a bandpass filter was applied to raw data with a frequency range of 20–500 Hz [5]. It is important to cancel the powerline noise, so a band-reject filter is used for the 50–60 Hz range. Figure 3 shows an example of raw data for each sensor.

The visualization of the signals acquired from each sensor was important in an initial stage but a more objective comparison between those signals should be attempted. Signal-to noise ratio (SNR) is a quite well-established parameter; hence, it was calculated through the ratio of peak-to-peak values of signals from muscle activation periods and of noise from rest period.

Table 3 shows the SNR values in dB for each of the three sensors and each of the gestures [6]. As it was predictable from the signals shown in Fig. 3, FSR and IR signals have a higher SNR than EMG signals.

2.4 Onset/Offset Detection

A crucial step for success in gestures identification is the onset/offset detection. The correct feature extraction from the signal requires a high precision in the determination of the time interval in which the muscle is active. Several methods

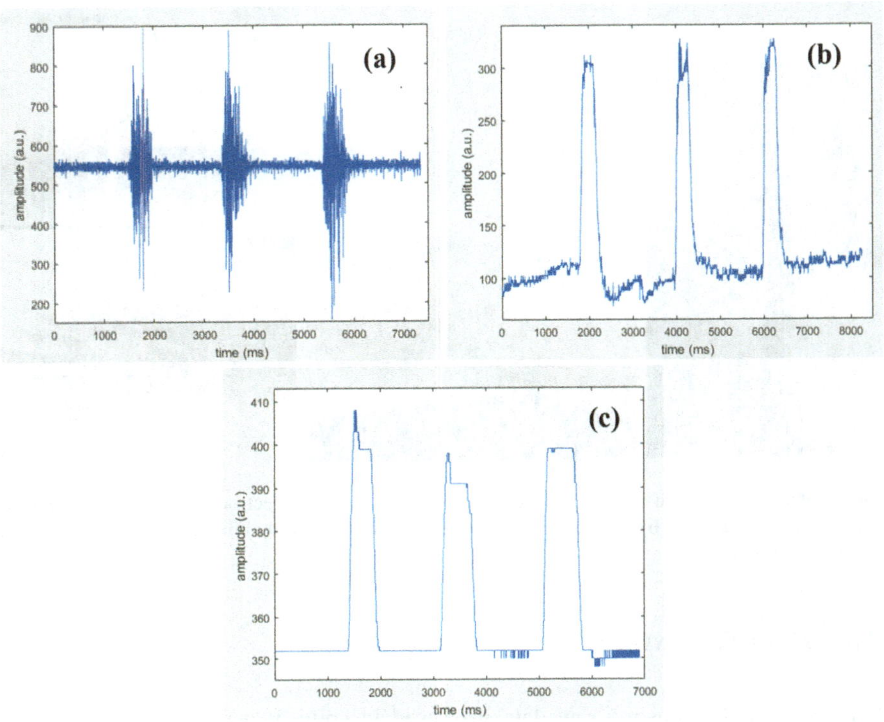

Fig. 3 Example of raw data of each sensor in case of a gesture of close. EMG (**a**), FSR (**b**), and IR sensor (**c**)

Table 3 Summary of SNR analysis

Sensor	Gesture	SNR (dB)
EMG	Open	4.5
	Close	2.1
	Point	2.2
FSR	Open	10.0
	Close	9.6
IR	Open	9.1
	Close	14.0

are available in literature [7–9], using different definitions of thresholds to find the beginning and end of a muscle activation, considering a single threshold of signal amplitude based on a deviation from the baseline of three times the standard deviation [7], or using a double threshold [8, 9]. Other method available in literature detects the muscle activity onset, using the energy of the signal, as it increases with the start of the activation [10]. In this work, the method selected for onset detection it is based on one proposed in literature [9].

The method used in this work for onset detection is based on one also described in literature [9]. It uses a double threshold with a moving average for calculating

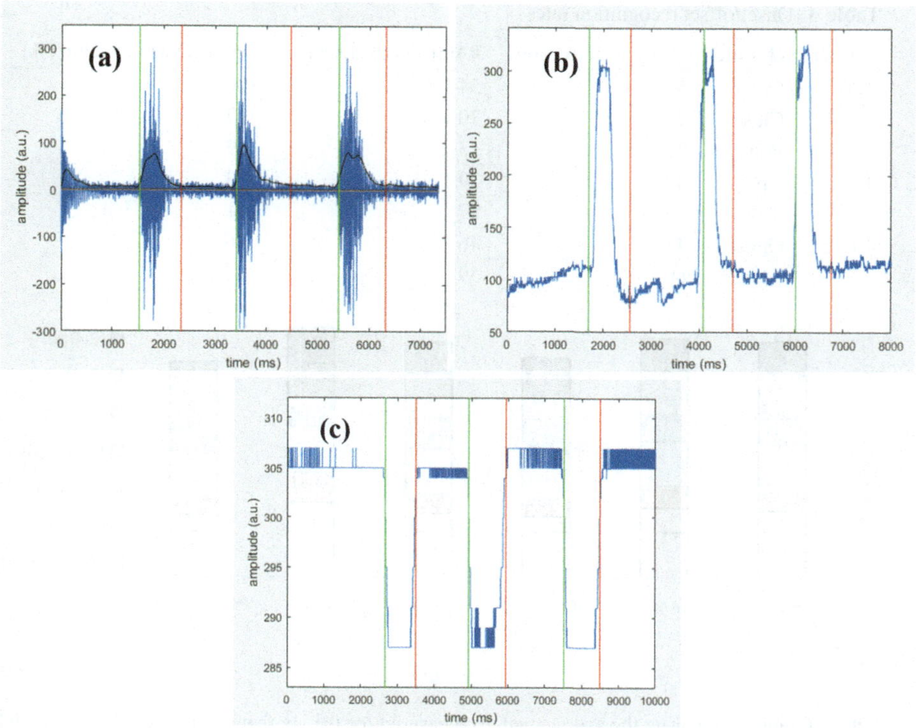

Fig. 4 Example of application of onset/offset detection in signals from each sensor, in case of a gesture of close for EMG and FSR, and open for IR sensor. EMG with envelope curve (**a**), FSR (**b**), and IR sensor (**c**)

an adaptive threshold. Besides EMG filtered signals, this method was also used for onset/offset detection of FSR and IR sensor signals; an example of its application in the three signals is presented in Fig. 4. Examples are the same as shown previously in Fig. 3 for EMG and FSR, and for the IR sensor it is an example of the gesture of open to show how it is distinguishable from the gesture of close.

3 Experimental Results

3.1 *Onset/Offset Detection*

The experimental data available from signal acquisition is different, depending on sensor and gestures as shown in Table 2. The main reason is the difficulty to maintain the correct placement of the sensor for every acquisition. These data files were discarded since it is not related to the sensor itself. Table 4 summarizes the onset/offset recognition rates for each sensor and gesture.

Table 4 Onset/offset recognition rates

Sensor	Gesture	#Muscle activations	#Activations detected	Onset/offset detection (%)
EMG	Open	54	54	100
	Close	72	70	97
	Point	39	23	59
FSR	Open	42	39	93
	Close	96	87	91
IR	Open	48	46	96
	Close	60	59	98

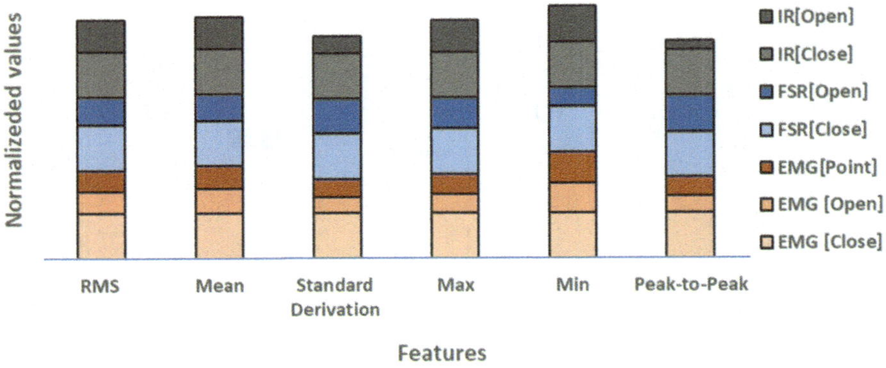

Fig. 5 Graphs comparing the average values measured for the six features in each gesture: EMG [Open; Close; Point]; FSR [Open; Close]; IR sensor [Open; Close]

3.2 *Features Extraction*

A set of features in the signal had been considered initially [11]. From the extraction of these six features in all of the data acquired in this work, it was found that just one or two depending on the sensor signals could be used for gesture recognition. This is illustrated in the graph presented in Fig. 5. The average values measured for the six features were previously normalized separately for each sensor and for each of the gestures considered; two or three gestures depending on the sensor.

3.3 *Comparison of the Success in Gesture Recognition by Each Sensor*

With the EMG sensor it is possible to detect signals of three different gestures, while with the FSR and IR sensor only two of those three gestures can be detected. From the average values of the features already shown in Fig. 5, different criteria had been

Table 5 Features and criteria adopted and percentage of success in gesture identification for each of three sensors

Sensor	Gesture	Criteria	Gesture identification	
			False/true	(%)
EMG[1]	Open	[$11<\mu<18$; $\sigma^2 < 6$]	6/48	89
	Close	[$\mu > 18$; $\sigma^2 > 15.5$]	22/48	69
	Point	[$\mu < 11$; $6 < \sigma^2 < 15.5$]	2/21	91
EMG[2]	Open	Other	9/45	83
	Close	[$\mu > 15$; RMS >16]	4/66	94
FSR	Open	[70 < RMS < 140; min < 40]	0/39	100
	Close	Other	13/74	85
IR	Open	Other	0/46	100
	Close	[RMS > 360]	0/59	100

established for the identification of those gestures. Table 5 shows the features used for each sensor and presents the criteria adopted. For the EMG sensor two sets of criteria were chosen: one for the recognition of the three gestures and the other for comparison purposes, with the other two sensors only the same two gestures were considered.

The results of the application of those criteria are also presented in Table 5 in terms of percentage of success, i.e., accounting the true and false events of gesture recognition for each sensor.

With these results a confusion matrix was built for each pair sensor/gesture and the analysis of these results had been based on the application of the well-known equations of generalized Precision, Recall (or Sensitivity), and Specificity [12].

As, in opposition to the other two sensors, EMG had shown capability for the recognition of three gestures, Fig. 6 shows solely its results with the purpose of evidencing the differences between the successful in recognition of each of the three gestures. Results are mostly between 85% and 95% with the only two exceptions of Recall or Sensitivity for close gesture (69%) and Precision for point gesture (54%).

On the other hand in Fig. 7, a comparison of success in gesture recognition for each sensor is presented; therefore, in this case, EMG results are reported to the recognition of the same two gestures as FSR and IR sensors. A very distinctive behavior is found for the IR sensor as it reaches the absolute success for the recognition of the two gestures, consequently achieving the maximum value on any of the three parameters. FSR and EMG sensors have very similar overall values of these three parameters but FSR with great discrepancy between the two gestures, excellent for open gesture but very deficient for the close gesture. EMG has a more balanced performance that is translated in also quite similar values of the three parameters for each gesture.

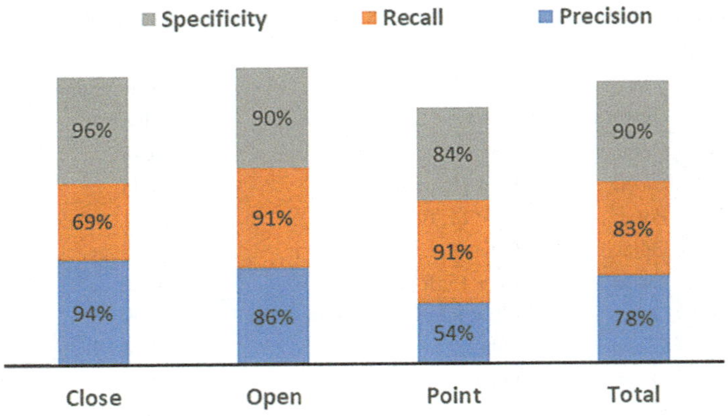

Fig. 6 Graph comparing the Specificity, Recall, and Precision for each gesture recognition using the EMG sensor

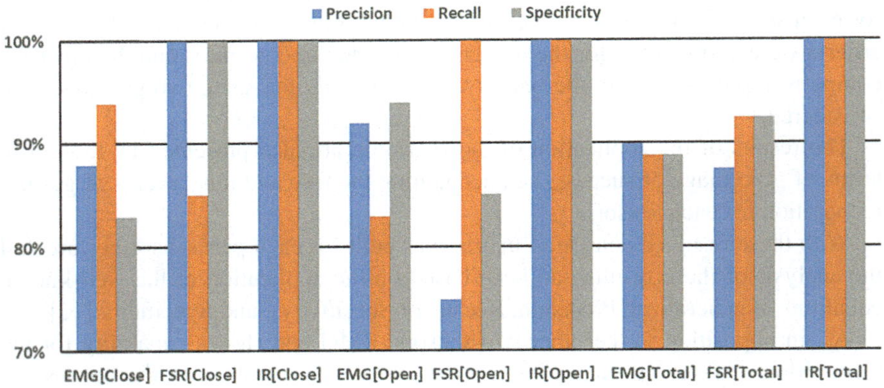

Fig. 7 Graph comparing the Specificity, Recall, and Precision for each of the two gestures recognition of the three sensors [EMG; FSR; IR]

4 Discussion and Conclusion

EMG sensors measure electrical activity of the muscles and are the more obvious choice for control hand prosthetics. However signals are often impaired by noise imposed by electromagnetic radiation and have low accuracy for finger movement recognition, as is demanded in bionic hands. A different sensing method may be more convenient, e.g., the use of force sensors to build a pressure distribution map of the muscle. But other types of sensors should be also investigated trying to measure any parameter that changes when different gestures are made.

This paper describes a comparison study embracing the application of an IR sensor besides the traditional EMG sensor and an FSR sensor, which has some results already documented in literature. IR sensors are able to detect movements in a muscle surface as its output signal depends on the intensity of light reflected by the skin with maximum distance of 6 mm.

Results from signal acquisitions of these three sensors had shown a slightly better ability of EMG sensor to detect different gestures, but simultaneously it has a lower success in gesture identification. IR sensors have shown similar results comparatively to FSR in the ability to detect different gestures but an even better success in gesture identification. Also IR and FSR signals had shown higher signal-to-noise ratios than traditional EMG signals, for the two gestures that those two sensors were able to detect.

There is plenty of space to improve these results from FSR and IR sensors, namely by the development of holders for a more solid fixation and placement. The application of a set of sensors instead of a single one is expected to highly improve the detectability as well as the specificity of finger motion recognition for both FSR and IR sensors. Also, some signal processing techniques can be applied, namely to reduce the effects on the signal derived from the poorly fixation. Further research should be carried out in order to find other type of sensors or combinations of sensors suitable for a more accurate gesture identification or finger motion recognition in modern hand prosthetics based on MMG signals/sensors.

References

1. Wei, G., Tian, F., Tang, G., Wang, C.: A wavelet-based method to predict muscle forces from surface electromyography signals in weightlifting. J. Bionic Eng. **9**, 48–58 (2012)
2. Li, N., Yang, D., Jiang, L., Liu, H., Cai, H.: Combined use of FSR sensor array and SVM classifier for finger motion recognition based on pressure distribution map. J. Bionic Eng. **9**, 39–47 (2012)
3. Keating, J.: Relating forearm muscle electrical activity to finger forces. MSc thesis, Worcester Polytechnic Institute, US (2014)
4. Xueyan, T., Liu, Y., Lv, C., Sun, D.: Hand motion classification using a multi-channel surface electromyography sensor. Sensors. **12**, 1130–1147 (2012)
5. Balbinot, A., Favieiro, G.: A neuro-fuzzy system for characterization of arm movements. Sensors. **13**, 2613–2630 (2013)
6. Papadopoulos, P., Tsiartas, A., Gibson, J., Narayanan, S.: A supervised signal-to-noise ratio estimation of speech signals. In: IEEE International Conference on Acoustic, Speech and Signal Processing (ICASSP), pp. 8287–8291. IEEE, Florence (2014)
7. Di Fabio, R.P.: Reliability of computerized surface electromyography for determining the onset of muscle activity. Phys. Ther. **67**, 43–48 (1987)
8. Bonato, P., D'Alessio, T., Knaflitz, M.: A statistical method for the measurement of muscle activation intervals from surface myoelectric signal during gait. IEEE Trans. Biomed. Eng. **45**, 287–299 (1998)
9. Silva, H., Scherer, R., Sousa, J., Londral, A.: Towards improving the usability of electromyographic interfaces. In: Pons, J., Torricelli, D., Pajaro, M. (eds.) Converging Clinical and Engineering Research on Neurorehabilitation, Biosystems & Biorobotics, vol. 1, pp. 437–441. Springer, Berlin (2013)
10. Rasool, G., Iqbal, K.: Muscle activity onset detection using energy detectors. In: Proc. of the IEEE Engineering in Medicine and Biology Society Annual Int'l Conf. (EMBC), pp. 3094–3097. IEEE, San Diego (2012)

11. Freitas, M.L.B., Mendes Junior, I.J.A., Pires, M.B., Stévan Jr., S.L.: Sistemas de extração de caraterísticas do sinal de TM eletromiografia de tempo e frequência em Labview. In: Anais do V Congresso Brasileiro de Eletromiografia e Cinesiologia e X Simpósio de Engenharia Biomédica, pp. 820–823. Even3 Publisher, Uberlândia (2017)
12. Sokolova, M., Lapalme, G.: A systematic analysis of performance measures for classification tasks. Inf. Process. Manag. **45**, 427–437 (2009)

Comparison of Different Polymeric Materials for Mobile Off-the-Person ECG

Daniel N. Osório, Alexandre Pitães, Nuno Gonçalves, Ricardo Freitas, Carlos Ribeiro, Ricardo Sá, Hugo Gamboa, and Hugo P. Silva

1 Introduction

Home health care has seen a significant growth over the recent years, with both an increasing interest by individuals in self-managing their health and an increase in preference for aging at home rather than in an institution [3]. This has been possible due to major advances in technology, increasing the availability of health solutions, which in turn helps patients to gain more flexibility, and helps physicians in the assessment of the health of the patient, providing insights into their daily life [1].

One of those technologies is the electrocardiogram (ECG), a measure of the heart's electrical activity. With cardiovascular diseases (CVDs) being responsible for a large percentage of deaths worldwide, proper monitoring of the heart by health professionals is more important than ever [4, 7], and recent studies emphasize the decrease in mortality due to prevention and acute care [2].

D. N. Osório (✉) · H. Gamboa
LIBPhys-UNL - Lab. de Instrumentação, Eng. Biomédica e Física da Radiação, Caparica, Portugal
e-mail: d.osorio@fct.unl.pt

H. P. Silva
PLUX - Wireless Biosignals, S.A., Lisboa, Portugal

IT - Instituto de Telecomunicações, Lisboa, Portugal

EST/IPS - Escola Superior de Tecnologia do Instituto Politécnico de Setúbal, Setúbal, Portugal

A. Pitães · N. Gonçalves · R. Freitas · C. Ribeiro
PIEP - Innovation in Polymer Engineering, Guimaraes, Portugal

R. Sá
SIOSLife - For Younger Spirits, Braga, Portugal

P. R. M. Inácio et al. (eds.), *5th EAI International Conference on IoT Technologies for HealthCare*, EAI/Springer Innovations in Communication and Computing,
https://doi.org/10.1007/978-3-030-30335-8_2

The placement of the electrodes used in recording this activity can be divided into three different categories according to their intrusiveness, namely: in-the-person, on-the-person, and off-the-person [6]. In-the-person refers to devices that are designed to be either surgically implanted,[1] placed sub-dermal, or ingested. On-the-person devices are those where the electrodes are attached directly on the body surface and are the most common type of devices. The least intrusive are the off-the-person devices, where the electrodes are embedded into objects, recording an ECG signal when the user interacts with them.

In the context of telehealth continuous monitoring, an off-the-person monitoring solution provides a frequent ECG signal source with low intrusiveness. There are already some devices on the market offering off-the-person ECG, focusing on embedding the electrodes on smart-phone cases, building some wireless accessories, or telehealth systems,[2] but these devices rely on stainless steel electrodes, which are difficult to embed.

This paper focuses on the evaluation of different types of polymeric electrodes to be used in a mobile off-the-person ECG monitoring approach. The usage of polymeric electrodes makes it easier to embed the sensors in end-user devices (e.g., a tablet or mobile phone), allowing the production of cases for different devices capable of capturing the ECG signal with relatively low production costs and in a user friendly way. In the following sections, a brief description of all the materials is presented, as well as the methodology used to perform the comparison between the different materials, ending with the results for each of the metrics used and a reflection about them.

2 Material and Methods

2.1 Polymeric Materials

In the scope of our work, different materials were tested, namely: stainless steel (SS) rectangles pads, used to get a baseline since they are widely used as a dry electrode in the state of the art; PolyOne's OnForce (PO), a polyamide with high elastic modulus and material strength; Vectra's 840i LDS LCP (LDS), a liquid crystal polymer modified to be used in printed circuit boards; LUVOCOM 1850-8023 PTB (LV), a polybutylene terephthalate polymer reinforced with carbon fiber designed to be electrically conductive; ET445 (CF), carbon fiber using an epoxy matrix; and RTP's 199 X 137556 E (RTPE), a polypropylene reinforced with carbon and stainless steel fibers designed for electrical conductive solutions.

---

[1] Medtronic Reveal LINQ.

[2] AliveCor Kardia Band and Kardia Mobile or Docobo Careportal.

2.2 Data Acquisition

To benchmark the different electrode materials for the purpose of ECG data acquisition, a biosignalsplux system from PLUX[3] was used. This hardware is capable of recording data up to 4000 Hz with a 16-bit resolution. For this study, a sample rate of 1000 Hz was chosen. A BITalino (r)evolution[4] ECG sensor was used, with the interface to each of the materials being done using metal alligator clips. This sensor can be used in a configuration using only two electrodes, a positive and a negative terminal, using a virtual ground to improve the common-mode rejection [5]. This configuration was used to simulate the assembly on a practical use case of hardware integration in a mobile device, which will have only two polymeric surfaces to record the signal.

To compare the usability of each material as an electrode, more specifically, if it was able to record a cardiac trace with medical grade quality, data from a clinical grade ECG system was simultaneously recorded. To this effect, a GE© MAC 800 ECG unit was used as gold standard. This system is capable of recording a 12-lead ECG with a sampling rate of 500 Hz, and exports the recordings in digital format as XML files (with a recording window length of only 10 s).

In [6], the authors state that the ECG signal obtained from electrodes placed between both hands correlates with lead I of the 12-lead ECG medical placement system. As such, out of the 12-leads, only lead I was recorded. The electrodes were placed following a typical Einthoven-triangle lead placement: one electrode on the right wrist and one on the left wrist. A third electrode, the reference (or ground), was placed in the right leg. A representation of the electrode placement can be seen in Fig. 1.

2.3 Experimental Protocol

To test the similarity of both signals, data was acquired simultaneously using the aforementioned setup using the following experimental protocol:

1. On the material in study, make a marking at 1, 2, and 3 cm from the electrode-alligator clips interface;
2. Place the MAC 800 system electrodes on the user, and verify the ECG signal;
3. Start data recording on the biosignalsplux software[5];
4. Ask the subject to hold the material at the 1 cm mark, wait for the signal from the electrode to stabilize (if possible) and record a 10 s window on the MAC 800;
5. Repeat the previous step for the remaining distances;
6. Export the data from the MAC 800 and change material.

[3]http://biosignalsplux.com/en/.

[4]http://bitalino.com/en/.

[5]http://biosignalsplux.com/en/software/opensignals.

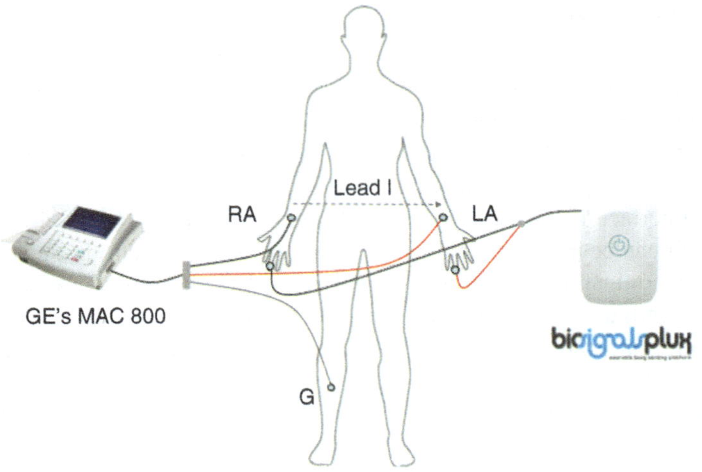

Fig. 1 Electrode placement for both signal recording systems. RA: Right Arm; LA: Left Arm; G: Reference/Ground

This protocol was used in four different test subjects, all of them males and with no reported cardiac pathology. Their mean age was 24.5 years with a 2.6 years standard deviation.

2.4 Data Processing and Signal Similarity

The first step was downsampling the biosignalsplux ECG to 500 Hz, in order to be compared with the ECG recorded using the MAC800. Afterwards, both ECG sources were time aligned. To that effect, the beat to beat pattern from the 10 s ECG of the MAC800 was matched to that obtained using the polymeric electrodes, with the R peak positions used to obtain the matching sequence. The R peak location was manually annotated. After synchronizing the signals, a digital notch filter with a cutoff frequency of 50 Hz was used to reduce power-line interference. Each source was then segmented by beats and each beat was standardized (Eq. (1)) and also normalized (to calculate the root mean square error, Eq. (2)), where μ is the signal average and σ the signal standard deviation. Figure 2 serves as an example of the processing stage output.

To compare the similarity of the signals, each beat from both sources was compared using the cosine similarity (Eq. (3)), root mean square error (RMSE, Eq. (4)), and Spearman correlation coefficient (Eq. (5)). To calculate the RMSE, the signal is normalized (Eq. (2)) instead of standardized. The cosine distance was used since its result is independent from the magnitude of the input signals, giving an output between [0, 1], with 1 being very similar signals and 0 very dissimilar signals. The RMSE gives a magnitude dependent signal, and therefore both inputs must be

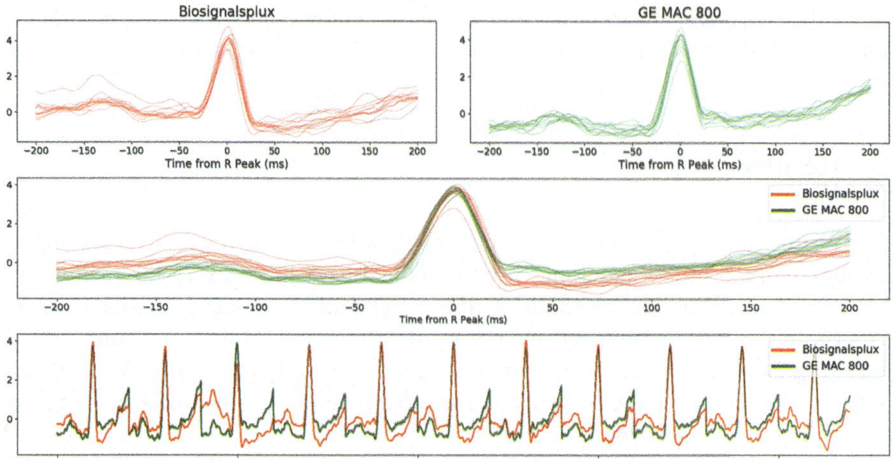

Fig. 2 Example of heart beat segmentation. Biosignalsplux signal acquired using LDS electrodes

normalized. This metric is an indication of the mean difference between both waves. Finally, the Spearman correlation was used to provide an alternative objective metric between the two waves. Unlike the two mentioned before, the correlation was used to assess the linear relation between them in addition to their morphological similarity. The range of results span from -1 (perfect negative correlation), 0 (no correlation), and 1 (perfect positive correlation).

$$x_{stand}(k) = \frac{x[k] - \mu(x)}{\sigma(x)} \tag{1}$$

$$x_{norm}(k) = \frac{x[k] - \min(x)}{\max(x) - \min(x)} \tag{2}$$

$$cos_{sim} = \frac{\sum_{i=1}^{n} x_i y_i}{\sqrt{\sum_{i=1}^{n} x_i^2}\sqrt{\sum_{i=1}^{n} y_i^2}} \tag{3}$$

$$d_{RMSEnorm} = \sqrt{\frac{\sum_{i=1}^{n} (x_{norm\ i} - y_{norm\ i})^2}{n}} \tag{4}$$

$$r_s = 1 - \frac{6\sum_{i=1}^{n}(rank(x_{norm\ i}) - rank(y_{norm\ i}))^2}{n(n^2 - 1)} \tag{5}$$

In Eq. (3), x_i and y_i are, respectively, the reference signal and the signal using the polymeric electrodes, with n the total number points. In Eqs. (4) and (5), $x_{norm\ i}$ and $y_{norm\ i}$ are, respectively, the normalized reference signal and the normalized signal using the polymeric electrodes, with n the total number points. The rank function is built in the correlation function from the Python SciPy library.

3 Results

The results for cosine similarity can be seen in both Fig. 3 and Table 1. Examining the box plots in Fig. 3 and Table 1, both PO and LDS have a very high similarity between the signals recorded using these materials and the reference, having comparable values to those obtained using stainless steel. In Fig. 3, a blue vertical line separates these materials from the remaining LV, CB, and RTPE. With LV, the similarity values are more inconsistent; however, the mean value using all subjects and all distances is still high.

Distance between the point of contact of the subject with the material and the sensor interface does not appear to play a big role in the first three materials, with their standard deviation being relatively small for each individual. For the final three, there is an increase in the standard deviation, with RTPE being the most affected by distance.

The results for the RMSE can be seen in both Fig. 4 and Table 2. The results for RMSE are in alignment with those obtained from signal similarity analysis, with PO and LDS having low RMSE and the remaining materials having a bigger and more scattered value.

The results for the Spearman correlation can be seen in both Fig. 5 and Table 3. Again, the results are consistent with the previous metrics; however, there is a higher dispersion in the results of PO and LDS when compared with stainless steel.

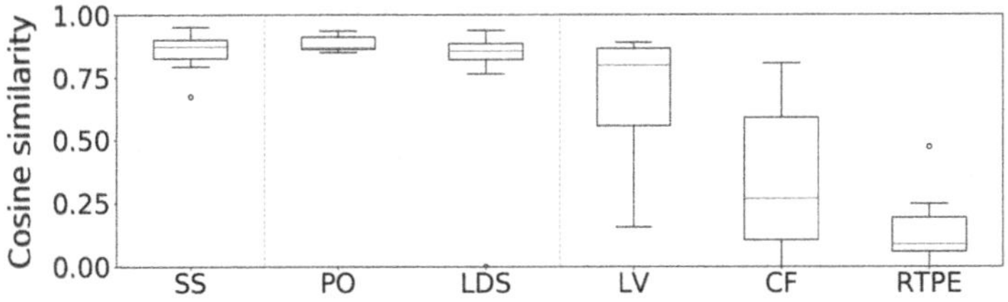

Fig. 3 Cosine similarity for each material. Values near to 1 represent more similar signals

Table 1 Cosine similarity values for each material and at different distances from the alligator clips

Distance	SS	PO	LDS	LV	CF	RTPE
1 cm	0.88 ± 0.06	0.89 ± 0.02	0.84 ± 0.07	0.66 ± 0.30	0.31 ± 0.34	0.16 ± 0.18
2 cm	0.89 ± 0.02	0.89 ± 0.03	0.87 ± 0.02	0.65 ± 0.17	0.38 ± 0.26	0.13 ± 0.10
3 cm	0.80 ± 0.08	0.88 ± 0.03	0.67 ± 0.39	0.79 ± 0.12	0.36 ± 0.27	0.10 ± 0.06
Mean	0.86 ± 0.07	0.89 ± 0.03	0.79 ± 0.24	0.70 ± 0.22	0.35 ± 0.29	0.13 ± 0.13

Values near to 1 represent more similar signals

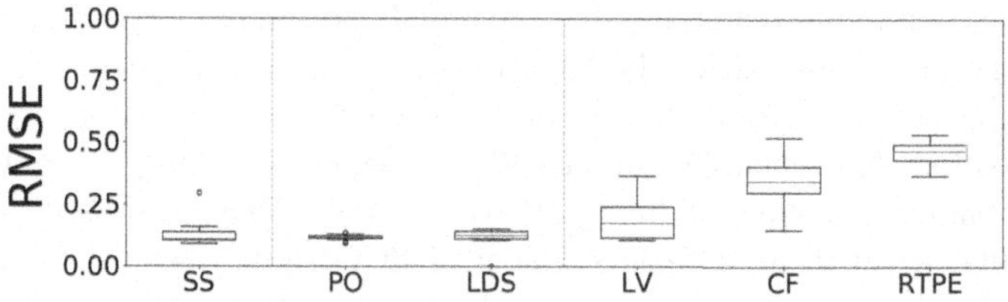

Fig. 4 RMSE for each material. Values near to 0 represent more similar signals

Table 2 RMSE values for each material and at different distances from the alligator clips

Distance	SS	PO	LDS	LV	CF	RTPE
1 cm	0.12 ± 0.02	0.11 ± 0.01	0.14 ± 0.02	0.20 ± 0.09	0.33 ± 0.09	0.45 ± 0.06
2 cm	0.11 ± 0.01	0.12 ± 0.01	0.13 ± 0.01	0.24 ± 0.09	0.35 ± 0.08	0.48 ± 0.04
3 cm	0.17 ± 0.08	0.12 ± 0.00	0.09 ± 0.05	0.15 ± 0.03	0.34 ± 0.13	0.47 ± 0.02
Mean	0.13 ± 0.05	0.12 ± 0.01	0.12 ± 0.04	0.19 ± 0.08	0.34 ± 0.11	0.46 ± 0.05

Values near to 0 represent more similar signals

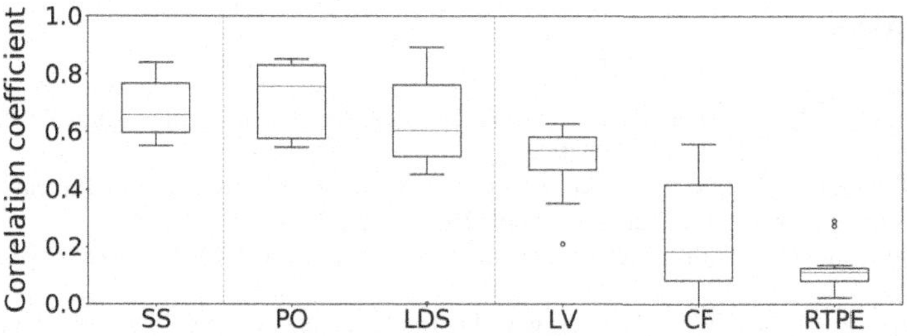

Fig. 5 Correlation for each material. Values near to 1 represent more similar signals

Table 3 Correlation values for each material and at different distances from the alligator clips

Distance	SS	PO	LDS	LV	CF	RTPE
1 cm	0.71 ± 0.10	0.73 ± 0.10	0.67 ± 0.13	0.50 ± 0.17	0.19 ± 0.24	0.15 ± 0.08
2 cm	0.71 ± 0.08	0.73 ± 0.13	0.67 ± 0.16	0.48 ± 0.08	0.29 ± 0.18	0.13 ± 0.09
3 cm	0.64 ± 0.09	0.70 ± 0.13	0.47 ± 0.30	0.54 ± 0.05	0.23 ± 0.18	0.08 ± 0.05
Mean	0.69 ± 0.09	0.72 ± 0.12	0.61 ± 0.23	0.51 ± 0.12	0.23 ± 0.21	0.12 ± 0.08

Values near to 1 represent more similar signals

4 Conclusion

The comparison between the different materials and a clinical grade ECG system revealed that stainless steel, PolyOne's OnForce (PO), and Vectra's 840i LDS LCP (LDS) is very similar to their respective clinical grade signal when comparing waveform morphology. Considering that stainless steel is widely used as an electrode, the results obtained for PO and LDS point to their possible use in this role.

By being polymeric materials, these materials are more easily embedded, e.g., in a casing of a mobile device. For the rest of the materials tested, the waveform morphology was very different, with these differences easily visible on the result section boxplots. For metal, PO, and LDS, distance does not play a significant role, with their standard deviations being relatively small. These results do not reflect the difficulty in gathering a clean segment of ECG signal. With the exception of stainless steel, PO, and LDS, it was very difficult to gather a 10 s window of clean signal, either due to the signal taking too long to stabilize or being impossible to record it.

Acknowledgements This work was supported by the Portuguese Fundação para a Ciência e Tecnologia (FCT) grant I&D 2015–2020 "iNOVA4Health—Programme in Translacional Medicine" (UID/Multi/04462/2013), and by the P2020 grant Senior Inclusive (NORTE-01-0247-FEDER-017967), promoted by HidePixel.

References

1. Artinian, N.T.: Telehealth as a tool for enhancing care for patients with cardiovascular disease. J. Cardiovasc. Nurs. **22**(1), 25–31 (2007)
2. Jarvis-Selinger, S., Bates, J., Araki, Y., Lear, S.A.: Internet-based support for cardiovascular disease management. Int. J. Telemed. Appl. **2011**, 342582 (2011)
3. Koch, S.: Home telehealth—current state and future trends. Int. J. Med. Inform. **75**(8), 565–576 (2006)
4. Mensah, G.A., Brown, D.W.: An overview of cardiovascular disease burden in the United States. Health Affair **26**(1), 38–48 (2007)
5. Silva, H., Lourenço, A., Lourenço, R., Leite, P., Coutinho, D., Fred, A.: Study and evaluation of a single differential sensor design based on electro-textile electrodes for ECG biometrics applications. In: Proceedings of IEEE Sensors, pp. 1764–1767 (2011)
6. Silva, H., Carreiras, C., Lourenço, A., Fred, A., das Neves, R.C., Ferreira, R.: Off-the-person electrocardiography: performance assessment and clinical correlation. Health Technol. (Berl.) **4**(4), 309–318 (2015). https://doi.org/10.1007/s12553-015-0098-y
7. Wilkins, E., Wilson, L., Wickramasinghe, K., Bhatnagar, P., Leal, J., Luengo-Fernandez, R., Burns, R., Rayner, M., Townsend, N.: European Cardiovascular Disease Statistics, 2017 edition, p. 192. European Heart Network, Brussels (2017)

Sleep Detection Using Physiological Signals from a Wearable Device

Mahmoud Assaf, Aïcha Rizzotti-Kaddouri, and Magdalena Punceva

1 Introduction

Sleep disorders are affecting a significant percentage of adult population, where insomnia, sleep apnea, and somnolence [18] are being the most prevalent. The lack of sleep has been associated with irritability and a negative mood, lack of energy and problems with memory and retaining information, and even weight gain and health issues. It has been recently shown that lack of sleep, besides resulting in lowered cognitive and physical performance is even linked to diabetes and cardiovascular diseases [16]. In addition, many chronic conditions such as diabetes, sleep apnea, and cardiovascular diseases actually result in an increased risk of an attack during sleep. Therefore new methods for detecting, monitoring, and managing sleep disorders are of essential importance today.

Physiological changes during sleep and sleep disorders have been extensively studied via polysomnography methods. Such methods involve collecting signals like the electroencephalography (EEG) for observing brain activity, electrocardiography (ECG) for heart rhythm, electronystagmography (ENG), electrooculography (EOG) for eye movement, and electromyography (EMG) for muscle activity or skeletal muscle activation. However, these methods are costly and require hospitalization of the patient for the duration of the procedure. Thus, increased research efforts are oriented towards a non-invasive monitoring of human physiological parameters as well as activity parameters. A wide range of wearable sensors are being developed for real-time non-invasive health monitoring, which opens up possibilities to follow sleep patterns and analyze the dependence between sleep and measured physiological variables.

M. Assaf · A. Rizzotti-Kaddouri (✉) · M. Punceva
Haute Ecole Arc Ingénierie, HES-SO, Espace de l'Europe, Neuchatel, Switzerland
e-mail: mahmoud.assaf@master.hes-so.ch; aicha.rizzotti@he-arc.ch; magdalena.punceva@he-arc.ch

P. R. M. Inácio et al. (eds.), *5th EAI International Conference on IoT Technologies for HealthCare*, EAI/Springer Innovations in Communication and Computing,
https://doi.org/10.1007/978-3-030-30335-8_3

Physiological variables of healthy individuals are controlled optimally during wakefulness to respond to the body's functioning. The body temperature, blood pressure, and levels of oxygen, carbon dioxide, and glucose in the blood remain quite constant and optimally regulated during wakefulness. During sleep, however, physiological demands are reduced and, for example, temperature and blood pressure drop. In general, many of the physiological functions such as brain wave activity, breathing, and heart rate are quite variable when a person is awake or during rapid eye movement (REM) sleep, but are extremely regular when a person is in non-rapid eye movement (NREM) sleep.

In this paper, we propose a method for monitoring sleep by use of physiological signals collected solely from a bracelet-like and sensor-equipped wristband which is comfortable, discreet, and non-invasive and therefore perfectly suitable for ambulatory settings. We collect physiological signals that correspond to electrodermal activity, heart rate variability, body temperature, and body movements. Our goal is to propose a system that objectively measures and estimates the periods of sleep and wakefulness, respectively, and we aim to achieve that by a machine learning classifier which classifies based on physiological signals solely. However, for training the classifier, we needed a labeled training set. For this purpose, we developed a mobile application that provides an intuitive user interface through which a user can register his/her sleep and wake hours while wearing the sensor-equipped wristband. The data provided by the user in this way are used to construct a training dataset which is further used to train a support vector machine based classifier. We show that by optimizing parameters of the classifier, we are able to correctly classify sleep and wakefulness in up to 93% of the cases. We present two applications, one implemented as a part of the mobile application and another on a cloud back-end application. We show that both types of classifiers ultimately achieve similar performance.

This paper is organized as follows: in Sect. 2 we discuss the related works, in Sect. 3 we present the problem formulation and our contributions, in Sect. 4 we present our data collection process, tools, and methods, the wearable sensor and the type of signals that we are able to collect with it, and the architecture of our system. We also explain our machine learning methods and classification results in this section. In Sect. 5 we present our mobile application and the user interface and we conclude in Sect. 6.

2 Related Work

Recent works related to ambulatory monitoring of sleep regularity focus on the type of sensors and sensing signals that can be obtained and the type of data analysis and the knowledge that can be extracted from the collected data. Furthermore, various studies focus on different types of sleep disorders among which the most frequent are insomnia or lack of sleep, somnolence or sleepiness, and sleep apnea [18].

In order to properly diagnose various sleep disorders, data regarding physiological signals are collected in hospitals via controlled laboratory experiments and this method is known as polysomnography (PSG). The polysomnography is the "gold standard" for sleep assessment [4], is very expensive, and can be intrusive to sleep itself, making the search for alternatives essential to the field. Study participants come to a sleep laboratory where multiple channels of data are collected. PSG provides general sleep measures, such as total sleep time (TST = sleep duration) and sleep efficiency (SE = TST/time in bed), light sleep (nREM1 + nREM2), and deep sleep (SWS + REM). The phases nREM1 and nREM2 are known as non-rapid eye movement and are providing measures of specific sleep stages referred to as light sleep, while REM, known as rapid eye movement together with SWS, known as slow-wave sleep, is often referred to as deep sleep. Polysomnography recordings include electroencephalography (EEG), electrooculogram (EOG), and electromyogram (EMG) of patient data among other signals [1].

In the last couple of years, the method known as actigraphy appeared together with the democratization and increasing usage of the non-invasive devices in many fields including health domain. With real-time information from the patient, collected in natural environment, this rich source of information allows users to change their lifestyle, predict and prevent hazardous events, optimize physical activities and sleep patterns [9].

Actigraphy is a non-invasive method, which can be used to infer sleep/wake patterns based on periods of activity versus inactivity, by analyzing raw data through specific algorithms [3]. The detection of movement is calculated by the accelerometer of the bracelet or by combining the accelerometer on the wrist with the accelerometer in a mobile phone. Actigraphy, in the domain of sleep medicine, has been a research method for studying a person's sleep-wake cycle, as demonstrated by the recent studies [11, 15].

There are three main actigraphy approaches [1] for inferring sleep quality: (1) objective approach based on measure metrics such as total sleep time (TST) and sleep efficiency (SE), (2) subjective approach based on self-reports via surveys and diaries, and (3) machine learning based, the approach that often combines the two previous methods, whose goal is to improve the objectivity and reliability of the observations from data collection via machine learning algorithms.

Sensor-equipped devices are being increasingly used to monitor patients with various chronic diseases, such as cardiovascular and neurological. Different sensors are combined and incorporated into wrist-wearable devices to be used in a plethora of applications providing feedback to users and also to health professionals. Currently, we observe a trend towards strengthening the customization or personalization of feedback to the users. In the domain of personalized health-care services [13] the evolution of sensor-equipped smartphones offers tremendous opportunities for monitoring. A variety of dedicated mobile applications offer new opportunities in psychological research [6] and many other areas. QuantifyMe platform [17] is one of the recent attempts that are starting to emerge in the quantified-self field. The goal is to allow to the non-experts to try to conduct self-experiments by use of appropriate methodology, in an automated way, using their smartphones. This technology is supposed to allow the users to find their personal optimal behavioral variables (e.g., bed time or physical activity) or to achieve their goals (e.g., productivity or happiness) based on evidence-based experimentation.

In a recent study [10] the authors outline platform aimed at processing physiological data from several wearable sensors and devices, namely Microsoft Band 2, Empatica E4, eHealth Sensor Platform, and BITalino (http://bitalino.com/). In this study critical comparison of the quality of HR and GSR signals is given. Most of the devices used in this study are wristbands, which are low-cost and accessible, thus creating opportunity for real life applications.

Several recent studies have compared the two most prominent approaches: polysomnography and actigraphy. In [15] the authors compared results for sleep monitoring obtained using PSG and the results from commercially available devices such as Fitbit Flex and Actiwatch among others. Different aspects were compared in this study: (1) regarding sleep efficiency (SE), it was shown that the device had low correlation with PSG, (2) regarding total sleep (TST), for all devices, a strong correlation with the PSG method was shown, (3) regarding light sleep time: significant difference with respect to PSG was reported, and (4) regarding deep sleep time measurements, the results were correlated with the PSG measurement. This study reveals strengths and limitations between actigraphy and PSG.

In [11] the authors evaluate the applicability of data obtained from a wearable activity tracker, Fitbit Charge HR, to medical research. This study was performed by comparing the wearable activity tracker, Fitbit Charge HR, with an actigraphy device, Actiwatch 2 (Royal Philips), for sleep evaluation and circadian rest-activity rhythm measurement. The findings of this study showed that the Fitbit Charge HR is a valid, reliable, and alternative device for use for sleep evaluations and circadian rest-activity rhythm measurements compared with actigraphy in healthy young adults. However, the sensitivity of the Fitbit Charge HR for accurately identifying activity was lower than actigraphy.

In [16] the link between electrodermal activity, skin temperature, and sleep was explored. They presented various feature sets for sleep/wake identification using electroencephalography (EEG) and actigraphy, while [7] elaborates more in detail about the EDA signal (phasic and tonic) patterns during sleep, and incorporates this information into a relatively simple method for identifying sleep and wake epochs using EDA data only. The results of this study indicate that electrodermal activity is not only a robust parameter for describing sleep, but also a potentially suitable method for ambulatory sleep monitoring. Automatic sleep classification based on support vector machine method and using EEG signal was presented in [2].

The heart rate signal for sleep monitoring was explored in [11] and [1], the reported results are encouraging but require complementarity with other signals. In [12] electrocardiogram (ECG) and heart rate variability (HRV) signals were used to classify sleep in infants and the correct classification reported was between 85% and 87%. In [5] different algorithms are used to predict sleep quality, using the heart rate and temperature signals. Our work differs compared to these works in the sense that it uses more comprehensive set of different physiological signals and their derived features.

The user interface and its different aspects and their impact on user together with practical considerations for designing have been discussed in [14].

3 Problem Formulation

Sleep regularity and disorders have usually been monitored and analyzed using polysomnography methods. Polysomnography is a comprehensive recording of the biophysiological changes that occur during sleep. A polysomnogram will typically record a minimum of 12 channels requiring a minimum of 22 wire attachments to the patient.[1] It is obvious that such procedures must be performed by a trained medical expert and require hospitalization of the patient.

Our objective in this work is to study and show to what extent it is possible to accurately detect the regularity of the sleep patterns in ambulatory conditions. For this purpose we use a wearable device that is equipped with multiple sensors and is usually worn on the wrist. The device is comfortable, easy to use, and poses absolutely no harm or risk to the user. Our contributions are the following:

- To the best of our knowledge we are the first to use at the same time, combined electrodermal activity (EDA), heart rate variability (HRV), accelerometer data, and blood volume pulse (BVP) together with body temperature in order to classify sleep and wakefulness. Previous works for sleep classification have concentrated on one or the combination of some of the aforementioned signals.
- We provide a study about various features and their relevance to the sleep classification problem.
- We have developed and presented a mobile application that is connected with the sensor-equipped bracelet to collect the physiological signals, provide data visualization and information about the regularity and duration of sleep patterns.
- We have proposed a support vector machine (SVM) based model to classify sleep and wakefulness, tested several kernels, and optimized the parameters such that the classification F1 score is up to 93%.

4 Methodology

Several wrist-wearable monitoring devices have recently appeared on the market among which the most prominent are Fitbit, Apple, Xiaomi, Garmin, and Fossil. However, the most comprehensive acquisition and access to raw data is currently

[1] https://en.wikipedia.org/wiki/Polysomnography.

provided by Empatica E4 sensor[2] and thus we decided to use it for the purpose of this study.

4.1 Wearable Sensor and Architecture

The Empatica E4 bracelet, the device that has been used for this project, offers the acquisition in real time of physiological data and provides full access to data for research purposes. The Empatica company has made available the Empatica Connect platform,[3] which allows to visualize the graphs corresponding to different signals. The bracelet works in two modes: (a) recording mode: the wristband records the data in the internal memory, and it can record up to 60 h. (b) Streaming mode: the bracelet connects via Bluetooth to the application.

The Empatica E4 bracelet is equipped with the following physiological sensors:

- EDA Sensor (or GSR Sensor): measures the fluctuating changes of certain electrical properties of the skin. It is measured in microsiemens.
- Infrared Thermopile: measures the temperature of the skin and gives the data measured in Celsius degrees.
- 3-axis Accelerometer: measures motion based activity, contains the data of the 3-axis (x, y, and z) accelerometer sensor. It measures continuous gravitational force (g) applied to each of the three spacial dimensions (x, y, and z). The scale is limited to $\pm$2g (by default) and can be extended to $\pm$8g with custom firmware. The accelerometer in our application is configured to measure acceleration in the range [$-$2g, 2g]. The unit is expressed in g which is 9.81 m/s.
- PPG Sensor (Photoplethysmography Sensor): measures the blood volume pulse (BVP) from which two signals can be derived: (1) heart rate (HR) and the interbeat interval (IBI). The blood volume pulse is measured in nanoWatts, heart rate variability HRV is measured in beats per minute (bpm), and interbeat interval is measured in time between two consecutive beats.

The architecture of our system is represented in Fig. 1. Figure 1 represents our system architecture. It consists of three main parts: (Subsystem 1) Machine Learning (top part, green-dotted rectangle) which aims at building the best performant model by iterating the different steps of the pipeline which are prepare data, extract features, evaluate and tune model, and finally build the best performant one. The final pipeline step consists of deploying the model on the repository S3 on AWS Cloud after being serialized. (Subsystem 2) Android mobile application (left part, black-dotted rectangle) whose aim is to interact with the Cloud Backend and make a Bluetooth connection with Empatica E4 wristband, gather values received from

[2]https://www.empatica.com/en-eu/research/e4.

[3]https://www.empatica.com/connect.

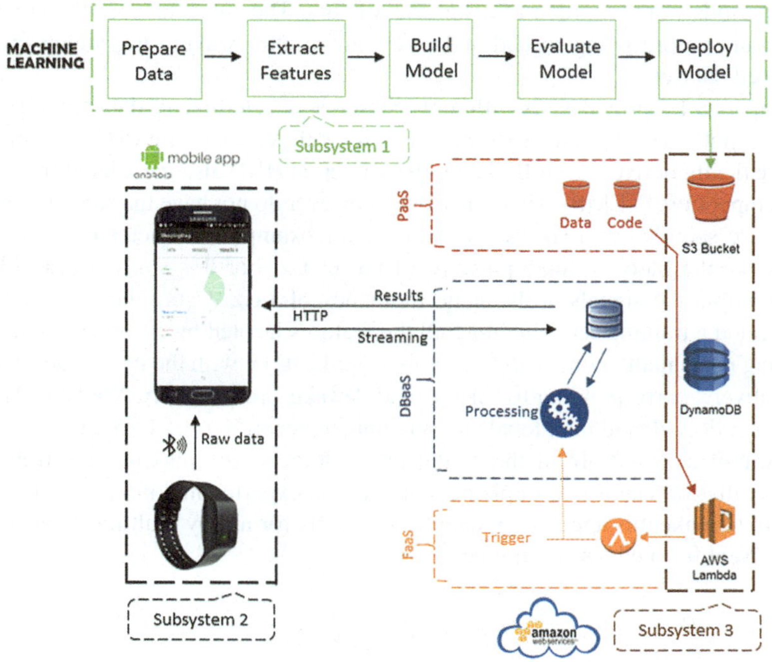

Fig. 1 Mobile application architecture

all the sensors embedded in it and sending them to the Backend. It also fetches the results from the Backend and visualizes them in a graphical and statistical way. (Subsystem 3) Backend and Cloud (right part, brown-dotted rectangle) composed by the three Cloud model PaaS (Platform as a Service) (S3 Bucket repository where we store some data and code), DBaaS (Database as a Service) (DynamoDB databases), and FaaS (Function as a Service) (Lambda Function where different Python scripts are triggered to execute many tasks like the prediction algorithm). The objective is to gather raw data received by the mobile application and sample them with a 600-s window. The prediction process is automated and launched after each recorded patient session and the results are stored in the dataset.

4.2 Data Collection

In order to collect data, each participating subject wore the Empatica E4 wristband for several days and for several long uninterrupted periods during day and night. Three subjects, two men and one woman, participated in this study. Each day they recorded the exact time of falling asleep and was recorded waking up. On some occasions, when they woke at night, such as going to the bathroom or drinking water, such periods were recorded as a wakeness hours. The subjects wore the bracelet a few hours before going to bed and a few hours after waking up, which favors a balanced dataset.

Empatica E4 provides six different measures: accelerometer data (ACC), blood volume pulse (BVP), electrodermal activity (EDA), heart rate (HR) (which is) automatically derived from BVP, interbeat interval (IBI) also calculated from BVP, and temperature (TEMP). These measures however do not have the same frequency, some are sampled at 1 Hz frequency like, for example, the heart rate (HR) and some like the blood volume pulse (BVP) at 64 Hz. For this study, we decided to downsample the signals at the same frequency of 1 Hz. Using the collected data, we created a training set containing all the features labeled by each participant. The labeling is manually done using the mobile application, with the two values 0 and 1, respectively, corresponding to "sleep" and "awake," respectively. We have 21 days of data collected, and the global dataset contains recordings of 1,058,374 s in total.

We collected data from three subjects as three is the maximum participants' number that we can use to implement and test an experimental model. In the future we aim to make this application openly accessible for use by multiple subjects with the consent from ethics committee.

4.3 Features Extraction

In order to better characterize the data collection, we summarized several statistics from the collected set of signals. We focus on measures such as the average values and the standard deviation in order to find out which are good features candidate for the classification algorithm. In the discussion below we summarized the measures related to a session whose total time is 15 h, 42 min and 16 s. The sleep and wakefulness period duration was 5 h and 18 min and 10 h and 22 min.

We have looked more in detail to discover how each signal is affected during sleep and wakefulness. In Fig. 2 we have represented the EDA signal for the three subjects during periods of sleep and wakefulness. Here we observe a significant drop when the sleep period starts and significantly increases when the wakefulness period starts. This observation is consistent with the EDA analysis in [8]. We

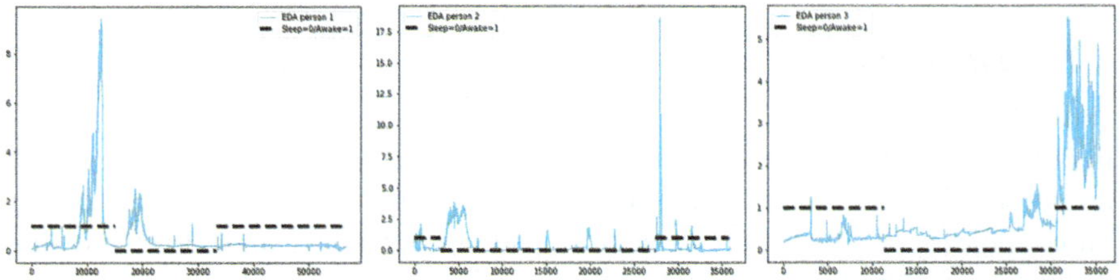

Fig. 2 Sleep and wakefulness EDA for the three subjects

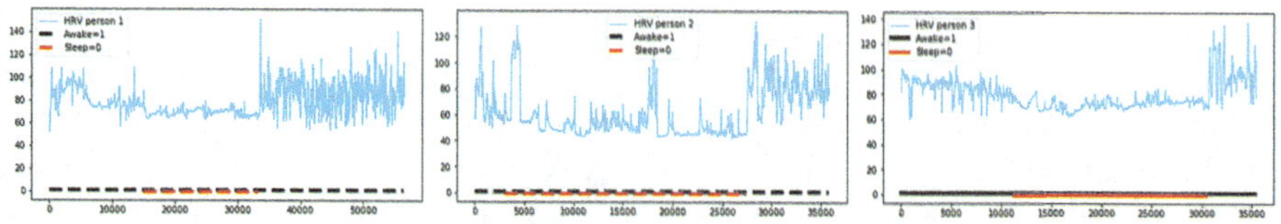

Fig. 3 Sleep and wakefulness HRV for the three subjects

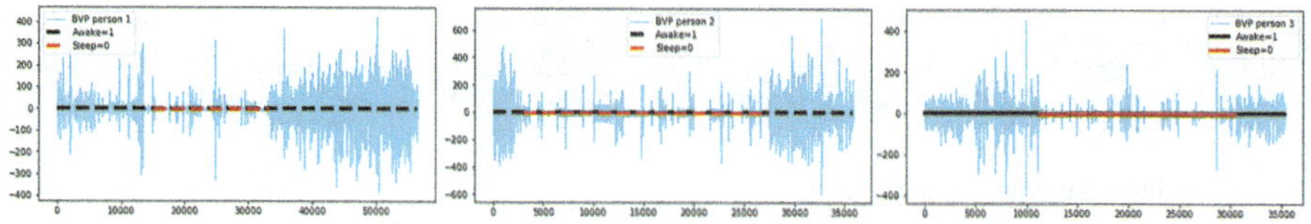

Fig. 4 Sleep and wakefulness BVP for the three subjects

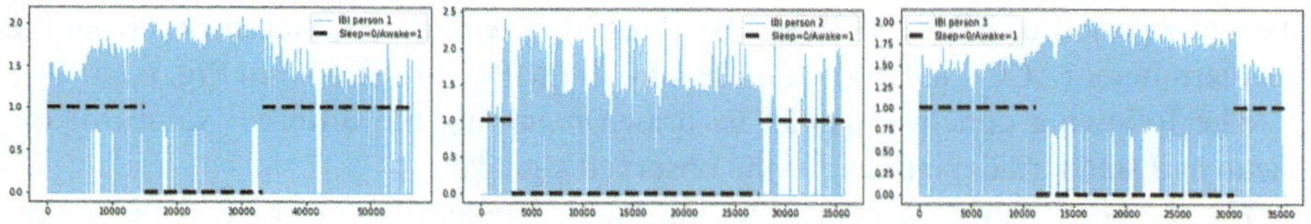

Fig. 5 Sleep and wakefulness IBI for the three subjects

observe differences between subjects, though. The drop in EDA amplitude at sleep period is more pronounced for subject 1 and the increase in EDA amplitude is more pronounced for subjects 2 and 3.

In Figs. 3, 4, and 5 we show the heart rate variability (HRV), the blood volume pulse (BVP), and the interbeat interval (IBI). As we mentioned previously, BVP is the directly measured from the PPG sensor and HRV and IBI are derived from BVP. As for the BVP signal from Fig. 4, we observe that the variance is significantly higher during wake periods than during sleep. This observation is consistent for the three subjects. Thus, the standard BVP deviation appears to be a good significant difference between sleep and wakefulness periods. Regarding HRV signal from Fig. 3, we notice that both the variance and the average values increase during wakefulness periods (compared to sleep), and this is also consistent for the three subjects. This is in line with the observations in [12] where the ECG signal is measured to derive the HRV for sleep and wakefulness classification and the average of HRV is considered as a feature for classification. As for the IBI signal, Fig. 5, we observe that its amplitude increases during sleep periods as the breathing slows down. This is consistent for the three subjects, as we notice that during the period of sleep the signal amplitude of the signal that represents the time between two beats gets longer. We see however that this feature does not improve the classification accuracy and shows that it can be omitted for the final classification without disturbing the performance. We discuss these details in Sect. 4.4.

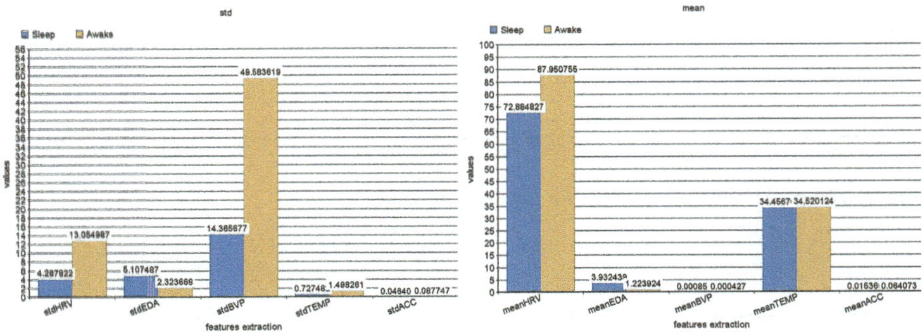

Fig. 6 Standard deviation and average

A summary about the values of average and standard deviation measured for the same period of EDA, HRV, and BVP together with the measurements from the accelerometer (ACC) and body temperature (TEMP) is illustrated in Fig. 6.

The following conclusions can be drawn regarding the different values of the mean and standard deviations for the observed signals:

For the HRV signal, when comparing the differences between sleep and wakefulness periods, the difference between the two average values is greater than the difference between standard deviations. Although the difference is not that high, we tend to choose the HRV mean as a feature. For the ACC signal, the difference between the two mean values is greater than that of the standard deviation; thus, we tend to choose the mean of ACC as a feature. For the EDA signal the difference in mean values between sleep and wakefulness is larger than that of the standard deviation; thus, we tend to choose the EDA mean as a feature. For the BVP signal the difference between the standard deviations between sleep and wakefulness is larger than that of the mean; thus, we tend to choose the BVP standard deviation as a feature.

We further built our model and tested the performance for separate features, doing optimization (tuning) and cross-validation for the training set. Some signals have shown a tendency to deteriorate the performance of the model, and that is why we did not choose them in the final model, TEMP and IBI. Finally we extracted the following features: average values for the heart rate (HR), the electrodermal activity (EDA), the accelerometer (ACC), and the standard deviation for the BVP signal.

4.4 Experimental Results

Our objective is to classify the collected physiological data into two classes, namely *sleep* and *wakefulness*, and for this purpose we have decided to use support vector machine (SVM) algorithms. SVM method has been already successfully used for classifying physiological data in other settings such as for classifying sleep and wake using ECG signal [12]. The SVM success is mainly due to the classifier's ability to create an optimal, highly complex decision boundary for the training data. SVMs use kernel functions to map the input space to a higher dimensional feature space. Optimization techniques are then applied to find the separating hyperplane that maximizes the margin between two classes in the feature space. This creates an arbitrarily complex decision boundary ideal for non-linearly separable data. We have thus explored both linearly and non-linearly separable approaches to investigate which one is the best for separating into the two classes sleep and wake.

Out of all the collected data, we created a training and a testing set by selecting 1764 records for the training set and 441 records for the testing set. The sleep and wakefulness periods were registered manually via mobile application dataset and serve as labels for the training set. Those labels were removed from the testing set. The features such as the mean values and standard deviation were calculated for a period of 1 s.

Next we tested combinations of selected features and performed fine-tuning of the SVM parameters to optimize its performance. We used scikit library to achieve tuning of the hyper-parameters of the classifiers. The library GridSearchCV exhaustively generates candidates from a grid of parameter values: when "fitting" it on a dataset all the possible combinations of parameter values are evaluated and the best combination is retained. Thus, using GridSearchCV we optimized the following parameters:

- Estimator object: in our case we estimated the best choice for the SVM kernel by testing the three options "linear," "rbf," and "sigmoid."
- Cross-validation parameter cv determines the cross-validation splitting strategy and the number of folds in stratified k-fold.
- c: penalty parameter used for the error term. Common to all SVM kernels, this parameter trades off misclassification of training examples against simplicity of the decision surface. A low c makes the decision surface smooth, while a high c aims at classifying all training examples correctly.
- gamma: kernel coefficient for "rbf" and "sigmoid." Gamma defines how much influence a single training example has. The larger gamma is, the closer other examples must be to be affected.

In our case the best value for cv of ten was estimated; thus, a linear, radial basis function (RBF) kernel and sigmoid kernels are used, and the optimal model parameters are determined using tenfold cross-validation of the training set.

We further tested and evaluated each signal with its mean and standard deviation to estimate their contribution value when used as inputs for the classification. We have observed that blood volume pulse, heart rate variability, and accelerometer data give fairly good classification results even when used as single feature. We decided to use F1 score to evaluate the classification methods, as F1 is usually more useful than accuracy in cases when there is an uneven class distribution, such as ours is. For example, we observe that the standard deviation of BVP, $std(BVP)$ with linear kernel gives F1 score of 0.82, the mean of accelerometer data $mean(ACC)$ with sigmoid kernel results in 0.93 F1 score, and the $mean(HRV)$ results in 0.84 when

Table 1 Classification results: F1 score

Kernel	Sigmoid	Linear	rbf
std(BVP)	0.81	0.82	0.82
mean(ACC)	0.93	0.92	0.87
std(HRV)	0.82	0.82	0.82
mean(IBI)	0.89	0.89	0.89
mean(EDA), mean(ACC)	0.68	0.92	0.91
mean(EDA), mean(ACC), std(BVP)	0.83	0.93	0.86
mean(EDA), mean(ACC), std(BVP), mean(HRV)	0.90	0.92	0.89

used with sigmoid and rbf kernels. We then combined pairs of these features and fed them as inputs to the classifier for each kernel type. The best result was obtained by combining $mean(ACC)$ and $std(BVP)$ with linear kernel, which resulted in 0.92 F1 score.

Finally we combined and tested sets of three and four features. The best results with three features were obtained with $mean(EDA)$, $mean(ACC)$, and $std(BVP)$ with linear kernel and that result is 0.92 F1 score. With four features, we have obtained 0.93 F1 score and the best results were obtained with $mean(HRV)$, $mean(EDA)$, $mean(ACC)$, and $std(BVP)$ with the "linear" kernel. As the HRV signal cannot be obtained directly via the mobile application the final combination of features that includes mean(HRV) can only be used through the cloud back-end application. Therefore when only mobile application is available for the purpose of training the classificator we can use $mean(EDA)$, $mean(ACC)$, and $std(BVP)$ without much deterioration in performance. For the cloud back-end application, in addition to these three we use $mean(HRV)$. These results are summarized in Table 1. In both cases, with three and four features, it is obvious that the best results are obtained using the linear kernel. This result holds for the two classifications that are with and without the HRV.

5 Mobile Application

Our mobile application communicates directly and collects the data from the Empatica E4 device and provides real-time information to the user about the regularity of his sleep pattern via an intuitive user interface. This application, developed for Android, allows connection via Bluetooth with the Empatica E4 bracelet. Using the application we are able to collect real-time data from the various sensors embedded in the bracelet E4, and these data are subsequently sent to the Amazon Web Services server where a database is stored, in order to make a machine learning processing at the server side. The application displays the EDA, BVP, and HRV signals for the user in the three different tabs of Fig. 7. This feature allows the user to observe the graphical representation of his vital signals and at

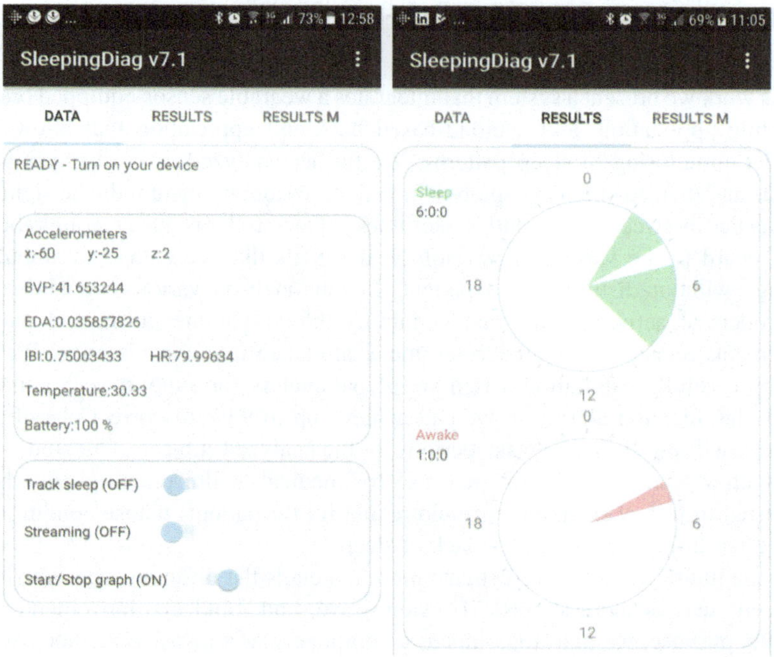

Fig. 7 User interface with a representation of the sleep pattern

the same time to make sure that the application works and that the signal values are successfully retrieved in real time. In order to save the battery and improve the application performance, a switch button "start/stop graph" is provided to start or stop the graphical representation in the background, when the display is not essentially needed. This allows to save the battery in critical periods. The results regarding the sleep patterns are displayed in a clock-like pie chart that represents the entire 24-h day data collection, Fig. 7. Using a spinner button, the user can select a date to view the results. The results are projected on two clock-like pie charts, the first in light green color is for sleep, and the second in pink color is for wakefulness. The periods that were not recorded and labeled are not visible.

In addition, the user has the possibility to manage application modes through other controls: (1) track sleep allows to start or stop sleep monitoring and control the data sending to the AWS server, (2) streaming: the "streaming" button allows to turn off the bracelet and stops the Bluetooth connection via the application. It also allows to reset the Empatica SDK to be ready to create a new Bluetooth connection. (3) start/stop graph: starts or stops the graphs display in the EDA, BVP, and HRV tabs, which saves battery and smartphone resources.

6 Conclusions and Future Work

In this work we present a system that integrates a wearable sensor-equipped bracelet, a mobile application, and a cloud-based back-end application that allows non-invasive monitoring of sleep patterns. We further analyzed a set of physiological signals and their features to explore which features among them indicate significant differences between sleep and wakefulness. Our study is fairly comprehensive with regard to the variety of physiological signals that we collect in ambulatory settings without disturbing the patient. In our analysis various signals such as electrodermal activity, heart rate variability, blood volume pulse, and patients' movements registered via an accelerometer are taken into consideration. We show that by carefully estimating a rich set of parameters for support vector machine based classification algorithm we can achieve up to 93% of correct classification when classifying sleep and wake periods for the analyzed subjects. Our study shows that such a system can be of great use for medical health practitioners who are interested to follow sleep patterns and regularity for patients whose condition is at risk either during sleep or due to lack of sleep.

In the future we aim to investigate more in details the different types and phases of sleep such as nREM1, nREM2, slow-wave, and rapid eye movement, REM. For this purpose, we plan to compare a completely non-invasive methods such as the method proposed here, with hospital grade quality sleep evaluation methods. Integrating user feedback about the mobile application is also planned as a part of our future work.

References

1. Alfeo, A.L., Barsocchi, P., Cimino, M.G., et al.: Sleep behavior assessment via smartwatch and stigmergic receptive fields. Person. Ubiquit. Comput. **22**(2), 227–243 (2018)
2. Alickovic, E., et al.: Ensemble SVM method for automatic sleep stage classification. IEEE Trans. Instrum. Meas. **67**(6), 1258–1265 (2018). https://doi.org/10.1109/TIM.2018.2799059
3. Anderson, W.M., Boehlecke, B., Claman, D., et al.: Clinical guidelines for the use of unattended portable monitors in the diagnosis of obstructive sleep apnea in adult patients. J. Clin. Sleep Med. **3**(07), 737–747 (2007)
4. Blackwell, T., Redline, S., Ancoli-Israel, S., et al.: Comparison of sleep parameters from actigraphy and polysomnography in older women: the SOF study. Sleep **31**(2), 283–291 (2008)
5. De Arriba-Pérez, F., Caeiro-Rodríguez, M., et Santos-Gago, J.M.: How do you sleep? Using off the shelf wrist wearables to estimate sleep quality, sleepiness level, chronotype and sleep regularity indicators. J. Amb. Intell. Human. Comput. **19**, 1–21 (2017)
6. Harari, G.M., Lane, N.D., Wang, R., et al.: Using smartphones to collect behavioral data in psychological science: opportunities, practical considerations, and challenges. Perspect. Psychol. Sci. **11**(6), 838–854 (2016)
7. Herlan, A., et al.: Electrodermal activity patterns in sleep stages and their utility for sleep versus wake classification. J. Sleep Res. **28** e12694 (2018)
8. Hwang, S.H., et al.: Sleep period time estimation based on electrodermal activity. IEEE J. Biomed. Health Inform. **21**, 115–122 (2017)

9. Kamišalić, A., Fister, I., Turkanović, M., et al.: Sensors and functionalities of non-invasive wrist-wearable devices: a review. Sensors **18**(6), 1714 (2018)
10. Kutt, K., et al.: Towards the development of sensor platform for processing physiological data from wearable sensors. In: International Conference on Artificial Intelligence and Soft Computing. Springer, Cham (2018)
11. Lee, H.-A., Lee, H.-J., Moon, J.-H., et al.: Comparison of wearable activity tracker with actigraphy for sleep evaluation and circadian rest-activity rhythm measurement in healthy young adults. Psych. Investig. **14**(2), 179–185 (2017)
12. Lewicke, A., Sazonov, E., Corwin, M.J., et al.: Sleep versus wake classification from heart rate variability using computational intelligence: consideration of rejection in classification models. IEEE Trans. Biomed. Eng. **55**(1), 108–118 (2008)
13. Li, H., Zhang, Q., et Lu, K.: Integrating mobile sensing and social network for personalized health-care application. In : Proceedings of the 30th Annual ACM Symposium on Applied Computing, pp. 527–534. ACM, New York (2015)
14. Liu, X., Ai, W., Li, H., et al.: Deriving user preferences of mobile apps from their management activities. ACM Trans. Inform. Syst. (TOIS) **35**(4), 39 (2017)
15. Mantua, J., Gravel, N., et Spencer, R.: Reliability of sleep measures from four personal health monitoring devices compared to research-based actigraphy and polysomnography. Sensors **16**(5), 646 (2016)
16. Sano, A.: Measuring college students' sleep, stress, mental health and wellbeing with wearable sensors and mobile phones. 2016. Thèse de doctorat. Massachusetts Institute of Technology
17. Taylor, S., Sano, A., Ferguson, C., et al.: QuantifyMe: an open-source automated single-case experimental design platform. Sensors **18**(4), 1097 (2018)
18. Zorick, F.J.: Patterns of sleepiness in various disorders of excessive daytime somnolence. Sleep: J. Sleep Res. Sleep Med. **5**, S165–S174 (1982)

Identification of IoT Medical Devices APIs Through Ontology Mapping Techniques

Argyro Mavrogiorgou, Athanasios Kiourtis, and Dimosthenis Kyriazis

1 Introduction

Advancements in wireless sensor networks have led to a potential interest in integrating data and capabilities provided by physical world objects into the Internet, leading to the emergence of Internet of Things (IoT). Therefore, as one of the fundamental constituents of the future Internet, IoT has attracted tremendous interests from various research communities and industries [1]. According to Machina Research [2], 27 billion of connected IoT devices are expected by 2024, while according to an analysis of Cisco [3], there will be 500 billion connected devices by 2030. Henceforth, it becomes clear that there subsist so many IoT devices around, and each day more and more IoT devices are coming into existence, resulting in a myriad of heterogeneous devices that are being connected to the IoT world.

However, in spite of its wide-spread emergence, IoT is still in its infant stage and has big room for research in variety of issues like standards, scalability, heterogeneity, integration with existing Information Technology (IT) systems, and so forth [4]. Among these issues, one of the most vital in IoT is the high degree of heterogeneity of the existing devices, in terms of having different specifications and functionalities. In such a scenario, it is necessary to manage the interconnection between such heterogeneous elements [5] that are expected to work in different ambient conditions and systems, offering their data. Therefore, the problem that arises is the difficulty of managing the enormous number of heterogeneous devices that need to be able to be connected in any platform that needs their data. Hence, it is of crucial importance not only to find out a way to integrate all these devices into different platforms, but also to find out an automated way to identify and understand

A. Mavrogiorgou (✉) · A. Kiourtis · D. Kyriazis
Department of Digital Systems, University of Piraeus, Piraeus, Greece
e-mail: margy@unipi.gr; kiourtis@unipi.gr; dimos@unipi.gr

P. R. M. Inácio et al. (eds.), *5th EAI International Conference on IoT Technologies for HealthCare*, EAI/Springer Innovations in Communication and Computing,
https://doi.org/10.1007/978-3-030-30335-8_4

their different Application Programming Interfaces (API), so as to be able to collect their data.

This requirement becomes extremely important in the digital healthcare domain [6], where IoT technologies have become a milestone advancement in this domain [7, 8], whereas the researchers have shown an increased interest in the sheer enormity of volumes of health and fitness data gathered from medical devices. Henceforth, especially in the healthcare IoT world, the need for communication among different devices is an issue of vital importance. Although a completely standardized system is an ideal solution, most commercially available medical devices include their own software and communication protocols, causing serious problems of heterogeneity, and thus producing an undeniable fact that each device works isolated and on its own.

To address this challenge, in this paper a mechanism is proposed for managing the huge amounts of heterogeneous medical devices that exist in combination with their derived data, by understanding the nature and the meaning of the API methods that can be found in these devices and are responsible for gathering their data. The latter is performed through a mechanism that initially constructs ontologies of the different API methods for both known and unknown medical devices, by identifying the different concepts and relationships among them. Afterwards, the mechanism identifies the syntactic and the semantic similarity between each different ontology and the different API methods that have been translated into ontologies. Henceforth, according to the mean of both syntactic and semantic similarity, the final mapping takes place, identifying the nature of the unknown medical devices' API methods. Finally, once the devices' API methods have been fully recognized, their data is gathered through an implemented generic data acquisition API, which is responsible for collecting all the devices' data. The proposed mechanism is evaluated through a specific use case, in order to identify the API method that is responsible for providing the medical data of an unknown activity tracker, comparing it with the API methods of two (2) other chosen activity trackers whose API methods' functionalities are known in advance.

The rest of this paper is organized as follows: Section 2 describes the study of the related work regarding data sources and data integration in the healthcare domain through the usage of ontologies. Section 3 describes the proposed mechanism for understanding the nature and the meaning of different medical devices' API methods so as to collect data out of them, whereas in Sect. 4, it is described as a use case of the proposed mechanism. Finally, Sect. 5 is addressing the challenges of the future internet, analyzing our conclusions and plans.

2 Related Work

Data integration is considered a key component especially in the healthcare domain, wherein most of the cases it is considered as a prerequisite in nearly every systematic attempt to achieve integrated care. In the context of healthcare, data integration is a complex process of combining multiple types of data from different heterogeneous data sources into a single platform, allowing multiple levels of users to access, edit, and contribute to their medical data [9]. However, without data sources' integration, their data collection becomes impossible, and if no data can be collected, no integration can be achieved among it. Henceforth, all these data sources should be able to be uniformly discoverable and integrated with different platforms, in order for the latter to provide access to their data, and thus giving the permission to integrate it.

For that reason, various IoT infrastructures have been proposed in the literature, especially in the healthcare domain, for addressing the aforementioned challenge, mainly based upon the usage of ontologies. In general terms, an ontology refers to a machine-readable representation of knowledge, particularly for automated inference [10, 11]. As a result, ontologies provide a sound basis for sharing domain knowledge between human and computer programs, or between computer programs, ensuring semantic interpretation [12]. An ontology normally defines concepts, instances, properties, as well as relationships, accompanied by their corresponding constraints [13]. Therefore, the power of ontologies lies in the ability to represent relationships between the concepts, whereas the main benefit of using the ontology-based models is their runtime interpretation [14], supporting the integration task that describes the exact content and semantics of different concepts more explicitly. Thus, semantic technologies in data sources and data integration solutions offer the abilities to represent relationships of data, relate data using datasets, and identify relationships for new associations [15]. For that reason, a lot of research efforts have been devoted into this area, where ontology-based models are used in numerous researches for solving both semantic and syntactic conflicts of heterogeneous data sources [16, 17].

To this concept, the authors in [18] presented an ontology-based architecture for achieving data integration within the context of the project presented in [19], where the emphasis was given to resolve syntactic and semantic heterogeneities when accessing integrated data sources. In the same notion, the authors in [20] proposed an ontology-based system, aiming to provide semantic interoperability among heterogeneous IoT fitness devices and wellness appliances so as to facilitate data integration, sharing, and analysis. Moreover, the presented framework in [21] defined a development process for integrating new data sources including their data description and annotation, by using the Ontology Web Language (OWL) [22], so as to model and describe these data sources. In the same concept, the approaches in [23–26] coped with the frequent modification of data sources' schemas, by providing homogeneous views of various data sources based on a domain ontology [27]. Furthermore, in [28] the authors proposed a semantic model for the description of smart objects using ontologies and description logics to enable semantic interoperability, while the authors in [4] proposed an IoT based semantic interoperability model to provide semantic interoperability among heterogeneous IoT medical devices. Finally, the authors in [29] described a process for constructing a suitable system to semantically integrate the data from heterogeneous data sources and ensure the interoperability of it, basing their idea upon ontologies, by using a hybrid method of ontologies architecture [30].

All of the aforementioned approaches propose several features regarding the integration among heterogeneous medical devices in order to collect data out of them, while all of them have identified ontologies as one of the basic technologies for the achievement of devices' integration and their data collection. However, none of these implementations uses methods for efficiently integrating heterogeneous medical devices of both known and unknown nature, thus containing known and unknown data collection API methods, correspondingly. As a result, all these approaches lack sufficient flexibility and adaptability to solve challenges arisen from integrating both known and unknown devices and gathering their data. For that reason, in our approach an innovative mechanism is proposed for integrating different IoT medical devices of both known and unknown API methods' nature, analyzing their APIs that are needed for the connection to these devices, and finally gathering data out of them. In order to achieve this, the proposed mechanism understands the nature and the meaning of the different medical devices' API methods, in order to identify and use the ones that are responsible for gathering the devices' data, and finally integrate it.

3 Proposed Approach

In our approach, a mechanism is proposed for understanding the nature and the meaning of the different API methods that are being used by different IoT medical devices of both known and unknown device type, so as to collect their data. This work is an extension of one of the basic steps of our previous work in [31], whereas it is oriented in the healthcare domain. In more details, the proposed mechanism has the ability to identify the similarities that exist among the different ontologies that are being created from different medical devices' API methods, not in terms of how does each method function, but in terms of what does each method represent and provide as a service. Henceforth, through this mechanism we are able to identify all the devices' API methods that are responsible for collecting devices' data, achieving finally their data collection and integration.

To this end, it should be noted that the proposed mechanism requires prior knowledge of the chosen medical devices' APIs (i.e., requested Uniform Resource Locator (URL) paths for accessing the APIs), while all the devices that are of unknown-type are being recognized as of known-type following the approach proposed in [32]. Consequently, all the devices that are being used in our mechanism are always of known-type (e.g., blood pressure monitors, activity trackers). Nevertheless, even though the devices of unknown-type are being recognized of known-type, their API methods' nature is still remaining unknown, meaning that we do not have prior knowledge of what does each API method is responsible for. However, for all the chosen medical devices (i.e., the ones of known-type and the ones that had unknown-type but have recognized as known-type) we have knowledge about (1) their API URL paths for accessing them, thus providing access to the different methods that are included into the APIs and are used for performing different actions, and (2) their API methods' descriptions. However, it is worth mentioning that the API URLs are not providing internal details to the end users for each different method in terms of their source code and their functionality purpose, but they are only providing descriptions on what does each method is supposed to do, when it should be used, and how it should be called. Finally, it must be noted that the descriptions of the API methods are usually provided in free textual format, but in our case, we are going to convert them in eXtensible Markup Language (XML) format, in order to use them as a basis for constructing the proposed ontology mapping mechanism.

In order to achieve all the aforementioned process, the proposed mechanism follows five (5) discrete stages: (1) the Ontology Creation, (2) the Syntactic Mapper, (3) the Semantic Mapper, (4) the Overall Ontology Mapper, and (5) the Generic Data Acquisition, as they are illustrated in Fig. 1.

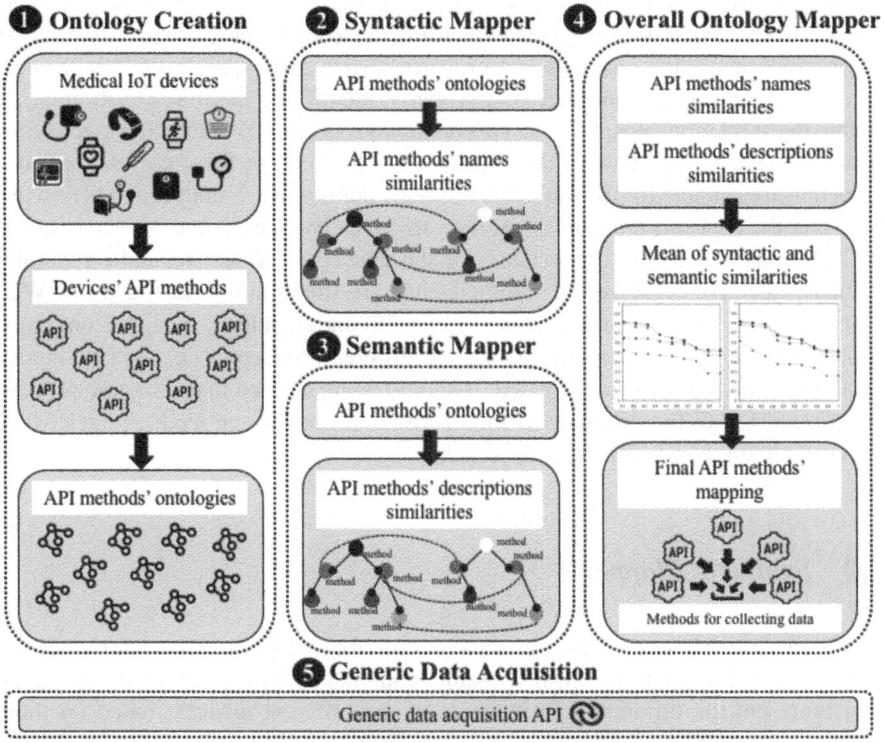

Fig. 1 Architecture of the mechanism

3.1 Ontology Creation

The Ontology Creation stage presents an automatic way for obtaining an initial organization of the concepts of the API methods from a collection of heterogeneous medical devices, representing them through ontologies. In more details, in order to create these ontologies, the mechanism implements three (3) different steps.

In the first step, the API methods of the chosen medical devices that are written along with their details in XML format are prepared for obtaining their concepts. To this end, the concepts can have super and sub-concepts, providing a rationalizing mechanism and property inheritance. In that case, the structure is analyzed to verify if the XML elements (i.e., API methods) have definitions that can be considered as concepts in the ontology. The elements are ignored if the structure does not have relevant ones; otherwise, they are considered to be included in the Ontology Creation process.

Afterwards, in the second step, it takes place the creation of the semantic relations for each one of the ontologies that will be created, referring to their properties, axioms, and constraints. To this end, two (2) types of properties can be defined: (1) the object properties that are related instances with other instances defining restrictions and behaviors, and (2) the data types properties that refer to properties that express only values. Regarding the axioms, these are used to provide information about the concepts and properties, such as to specify the relationship of two (2) concepts or the range of a property, identifying possible constraints. To define these relationships, the concepts are analyzed using WordNet [33], verifying possible correlations between the considered concepts. For these correlations, the ones that are suitable for the use in the ontology definition are analyzed, wherein the case that the concepts are synonyms, they are given an equivalence defined axiom.

In the third step, the organization of the concepts and the semantic relations occurs, which are organized in ontologies that are stored in files encoded in OWL. Consequently, using all the obtained concepts and relations, a single ontology describing the entire hierarchy among the different concepts (i.e., API methods) of a single medical device is created. It should be mentioned that the same process is repeated for all the different API methods of all the chosen medical devices, in order to obtain their ontological structure.

3.2 Syntactic Mapper

The Syntactic Mapper stage provides a way for mapping and identifying the syntactic similarity among all the possible combinations of the created ontologies that represent the different API methods of the different devices, based on their syntactic form. The goal of this stage is to identify the similarity measure among the different created ontologies, and provide the probability that a specific ontology is the same—in terms of its syntactic interpretation—with another ontology, mainly referring to the ontologies that belong to the medical devices for whom we do not have any prior knowledge about their API methods' nature, and we are looking for their API methods that are responsible for collecting their data. In our case, in order to measure the syntactic similarity between the created ontologies, four (4) discrete steps are followed.

In the first step, the identification of the ontologies occurs, whose syntactic similarity is measured. In more details, the Syntactic Mapper automatically identifies and iterates over each different ontology that has been created from the previous stage (i.e., Ontology Creation) and provides each ontology as an input to the mechanism.

In the second step, the transformation of the syntactical representation of the ontologies to their upper case characters occurs, which are then split up into different character groups, in order for their interpretation to make sense and being readable (e.g., getActivityToday() is split up into {GET, ACTIVITY, TODAY}). Shortly, this part iterates over the syntactical form of each created ontology, and identifies word patterns—in terms of words that are frequently met and repeated. As soon as these patterns are identified, they are split and stored into different tables for each ontology, resulting in the identification of the different character groups that are met.

Therefore, in the third step, the checking of the multiple character groups takes place, in order to identify which characters can be found in the split strings. In more details, this part of the Syntactic Mapper iterates over each different identified group, and finds for each ontology all the groups that have exact match with a different group. Hence, the outcome of this step is the total different character groups that are similar among the compared ontologies.

Finally, in the fourth step, the identification of the probability of resemblance (i.e., similarity) according to formula (1) occurs, indicating how much a specific ontology is syntactically the same with another ontology. Shortly, the syntactic similarity between two (2) given ontologies $C1$ and $C2$ is twice the number of character groups that are common to both strings, divided by the sum of the number of the character groups that are identified in both ontologies. Therefore, this step is iteratively followed for all the different combinations that can be constructed among the different created ontologies, in order to calculate their syntactic similarity.

$$\text{Similarity} = \frac{2 * (\text{CharacterGroups}\ (C1) \cap \text{CharacterGroups}\ (C2))}{(\text{Characters}\ (C1) + \text{Characters}\ (C2))} \tag{1}$$

3.3 *Semantic Mapper*

The Semantic Mapper stage provides the means for aligning and mapping the different ontologies, according to their semantical meaning. This process involves running several mapping operations, according to the resemblance between the created ontologies, and then filtering their results so as to find an overall alignment.

Once aligned, a direct connection or mapping is made among the created ontologies. In the case of the Semantic Mapper, the semantic matches between ontologies are based on the relationships and dependencies between their names' structures, and placement of instances. Therefore, in our mechanism, since the API methods are only providing descriptions on what does each method do, when it should be used and how it should be called, these three (3) criteria are used for identifying the semantic similarities between the created ontologies. In more details, in order to measure the semantic similarity between the created ontologies, two (2) different steps are followed.

In the first step, the identification of the similarity that exists between the created ontologies and is related with the aforementioned criteria for each method takes place, by utilizing semantic approaches that aim at identifying similarities between the semantical meaning of the API methods. In our case, Natural Language Process (NLP) semantic analysis [34] is performed so as to understand the semantic meaning of an API method's description. In that case, an Artificial Neural Network (ANN) has been constructed [35], based on the Multiple Layer Feed-Forward Neural Network (MLFFN) algorithm [36], whereas in order to identify the possible error in the translation of the semantic meaning of the API method description, the adopted error metric is calculated [37]. More particularly, this metric refers to the mean squared error (*E*) between output (Oi) and desired correct output (Ci), divided by the total number of the API methods' descriptions (*n*), as stated in formula (2). Thus, the specific ANN identifies the semantical meaning of the description of each API method, and probabilistically matches the different ontologies between the medical devices for whom we have prior knowledge about its API methods' nature, and the medical devices for whom we do not have any prior knowledge about its API methods' nature.

$$E = \frac{1}{n}\sum\nolimits_{i=1}^{\infty} (\mathrm{Ci} - \mathrm{Oi})^2 \qquad (2)$$

In the next step, the identification of the semantic similarity between the ontologies occurs, and it is calculated in the case that the created ontologies have common members or relationships. In that scenario, the same algorithm is implemented, probabilistically mapping the different ontologies based on their relationships. By the time that these steps are performed for each different ontology, different probabilities of the correspondence between the multiple ontologies are provided. As soon as the mapping between the semantic meanings of the different ontologies has been performed, the metrics of the final results' precision and recall are identified, so as to finally calculate the harmonic mean (F_{measure}) of these measures, with respect to the Unified Medical Language System (UMLS) reference alignment [38]. In more details, the following metrics are calculated:

- The precision that refers to the fraction of the retrieved data that are relevant to the query, displaying the number of correct results, divided by the number of all returned results (3).

$$\text{Precision} = \frac{(\text{RelevantData} \cap \text{RetrievedData})}{\text{RetrievedData}} \tag{3}$$

- The recall that refers to the fraction of the relevant data that are retrieved, displaying the number of correct results, divided by the number of results that should have been returned (4).

$$\text{Recall} = \frac{(\text{RelevantData} \cap \text{RetrievedData})}{\text{RelevantData}} \tag{4}$$

- The F_{measure} that refers to the harmonic mean of the precision and the recall (5).

$$F_{\text{measure}} = \frac{2 * (\text{Precision} * \text{Recall})}{(\text{Precision} + \text{Recall})} \tag{5}$$

Henceforth, F_{measure} is finally providing the number that indicates how much a specific ontology is semantically the same with another ontology. By the time that the Semantic Mapper finishes this process, the overall mapping results are stored, and provided along with Syntactic Mapper's results, to the next stage (i.e., Overall Ontology Mapper).

3.4 Overall Ontology Mapper

The Overall Ontology Mapper stage provides a way for aggregating and merging the results that have derived from the previous stages (i.e., Syntactic Mapper and Semantic Mapper), so as to finally identify the meaning and the nature of the API methods of unknown nature. Thus, the goal of this stage is to find the API methods' overall similarities, following two (2) sequential steps.

Firstly, the Overall Ontology Mapper queries through the syntactic and semantic similarity values that have been calculated for each different combination of ontologies, and provides a mean between them. This mean is calculated as the total of the syntactic similarity and the F_{measure}, divided by two, as presented in formula (6).

$$\text{Mean} = \frac{\text{Similarity} + F_{\text{measure}}}{2} \tag{6}$$

In the next step, the final identification of the ontologies of the API methods of unknown nature occurs. In more details, according to the mean of the syntactic and the semantic similarity that was calculated, an ontology is characterized that it matches to a specific API method in the case that it is over the threshold of 0.9 (i.e., 90% syntactic and semantic similarity). In the case that the mean is lower that this threshold, then the API method with higher probability of similarity automatically considers that it represents the specific ontology. This mechanism iterates for all the created ontologies, so as to finally identify all the API methods of unknown nature. Henceforth, through this way, we are able to extract the API methods that are responsible for collecting data out of the corresponding medical devices, which is the primary goal of our mechanism.

3.5 Generic Data Acquisition

In the Generic Data Acquisition stage, as soon as all the API methods for gathering data have been identified, the implementation of the generic data acquisition API occurs. More particularly, the latter constitutes a unified API that merges into a single unified data method all the different medical devices' API methods that are responsible for collecting their data. Thus, this API is responsible for finally collecting the data from all the chosen medical devices. It should be mentioned that after each iteration of the mechanism, the generic data acquisition API is dynamically updated based upon all the existing API methods, covering a wider range of methods and medical devices. To this end, if during the testing it is observed that the developed API does not meet the expected results, a feedback loop to the Syntactic Mapper takes place in order to cope with potential inefficient and incomplete results that may have occurred.

4 Use Case Description

4.1 Use Case Description

The use case exploits three (3) different IoT medical devices that have been already classified into the category of activity trackers, for which there exists only information about the API methods' nature of the two (2) devices, which are the Fitbit and the iHealth activity trackers. In more details, for these two (2) chosen devices, we have knowledge about their provided API methods in terms of how they are called (i.e., requested URL path), and what they offer as functionality (i.e., general description), as shown in Table 1.

In order to evaluate the efficiency of the proposed mechanism, an additional medical device is used, for which there is not any information apart from the API methods that it provides, in terms of how they are called (i.e., requested URL path), what they offer as functionality (i.e., general description), and the fact that this device is a Misfit activity tracker (Table 2). However, concerning the general description of this device's API methods, even though we have the syntactic description of it, we do not know the exact semantic meaning of it, in contrast to the descriptions of the Fitbit and iHealth API methods' general descriptions, whose both

Table 1 Information of the known devices API methods

Method identifier	Requested URL path	General description
Fitbit	https://api.fitbit.com/1/user/[user-id]/...	
FIT1	activities/date/[date].json	Daily activity summary
FIT2	[resource-path]/date/[date]/[period].json	Activity time series
FIT3	[resource-path]/date/[date]/[date]/[detail-level].json	Activity intraday time series
FIT4	activities/list.json	Activity logs list
FIT5	activities/[activity-id].json	Activity type
FIT6	activities/frequent.json	Frequent activities
FIT7	activities/recent.json	Recent activity types
FIT8	activities/favorite.json	Favorite activities
FIT9	activities/goals/[period].json	Activity goals
iHealth	https://api.ihealthlabs.com:8443/openapiv2/user/user-id/...	
ihealth1	activity/	Data of activity report
ihealth2	application/activity/	All activity report data

Table 2 Information of the unknown devices API methods

Method identifier	Requested URL path	General description
Unknown	https://api.misfitwearables.com/move/resource/v1/user/:userId/...	
Unknown1	activity/goals?start_date=X&end_date=Y	Goals in the period
Unknown2	activity/summary?start_date=X&end_date=Y&detail=true	Summary of activity in the period
Unknown3	activity/sessions?start_date=X&end_date=Y	Sessions in the range

syntactic and semantic meanings are known in advance. Therefore, the main goal of this mechanism is to identify the API method that is responsible for providing and gathering the medical data of the Misfit activity tracker, comparing it one-by-one with the API methods of the Fitbit and the iHealth devices.

4.2 Experimental Results

The proposed mechanism was developed in Java SE using the NetBeans IDE v8.0.2 [39], and ran in a Windows Laptop with an Intel Core i7-4600U CPU @ 2.10 GHz × 4, allocating 8 GB of RAM. Concerning the results of the mechanism, these are depicted below, following the five (5) stages explained in Sect. 3.

Ontology Creation In this stage, the hierarchical trees of the API methods were created (Figs. 2, 3, and 4) representing the classes (i.e., API methods' identifiers),

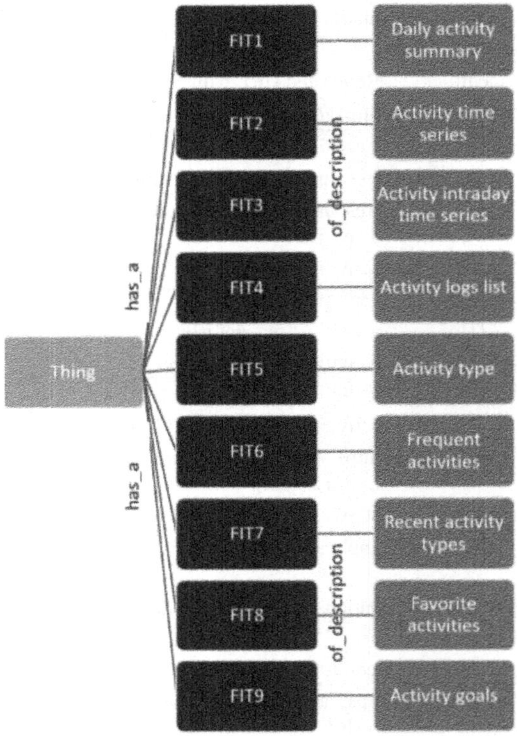

Fig. 2 Ontologies of the API methods of the Fitbit medical device

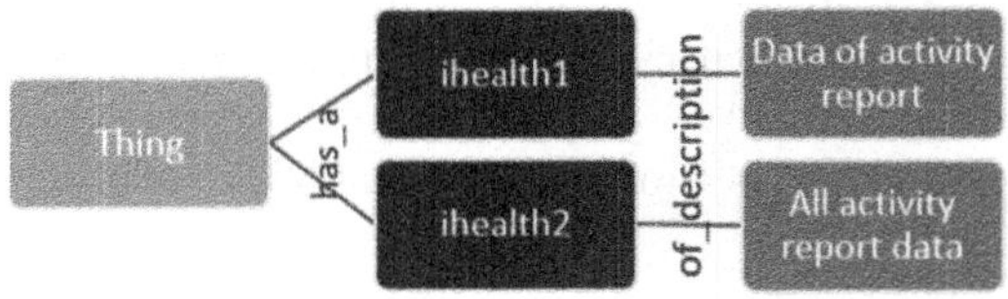

Fig. 3 Ontologies of the API methods of the iHealth medical device

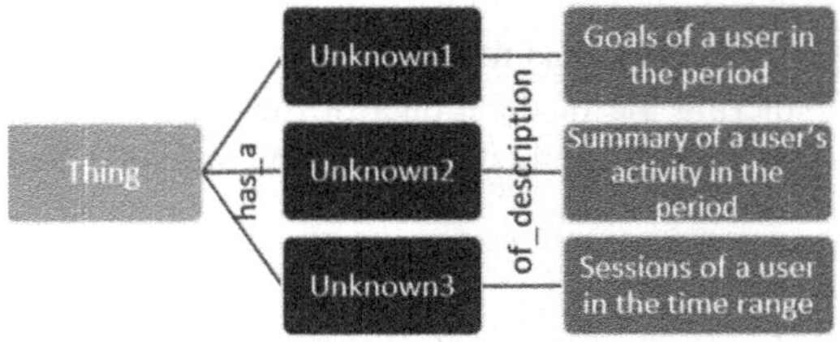

Fig. 4 Ontologies of the API methods of the unknown medical device

relationships, and instances (i.e., methods' descriptions), for the three (3) activity trackers.

Syntactic Mapper In sequel, in this stage, a syntactic comparison between all the different API methods—that are being accessed through the given requested URL paths—was performed, resulting in Table 3 that depicts a snapshot of the top-1 API methods of the two (2) known activity trackers that had the greatest values

Table 3 Syntactic mapper results

Unknown device	Fitbit device	iHealth device
Method identifier	Method (URL path) similarity	Method (URL path) similarity
Unknown1	*FIT9* 98%	*ihealth1* 33%
Unknown2	*FIT1* 86%	*ihealth1* 33%
Unknown3	*FIT8* 53%	*ihealth1* 33%

Table 4 Semantic mapper results

Unknown device	Fitbit device	iHealth device
Method identifier	Method (description) similarity	Method (description) similarity
Unknown1	*FIT9* 100%	*ihealth2* 89%
Unknown2	*FIT1* 95%	*ihealth1* 73%
Unknown3	*FIT4* 52%	*ihealth1* 99%

Table 5 Overall ontology mapper results

Unknown device	Fitbit device	iHealth device
Method identifier	Overall method similarity	Overall method similarity
Unknown1	*FIT9* 99%	*ihealth2* 89%
Unknown2	*FIT1* 90.5%	*ihealth1* 53%
Unknown3	*FIT4* 52%	*ihealth1* 66%

of syntactic similarity (i.e., similarity) among the API methods of the Misfit activity tracker.

Semantic Mapper Sequentially, in this stage, a semantic comparison among all the different API methods' general descriptions was performed, resulting in Table 4 that depicts a snapshot of the top-1 API methods of the two (2) known activity trackers that had the greatest values of semantic similarity (i.e., F_{measure}) among the API methods of the Misfit activity tracker.

Overall Ontology Mapper Finally, after successfully performing all the aforementioned tasks, the calculated means of the Syntactic and the Semantic Mapper results were merged, providing finally the API methods of the Misfit activity tracker with higher probabilities of resemblance with the other API methods (i.e., Fitbit and iHealth), in order to understand their meaning (*highlighted with gray color*), and identify the API method of the Misfit activity tracker that was finally able to gather its medical data. Consequently, according to Table 5:

- The *Unknown1* method was used for getting the activity goals.
- The *Unknown2* method was used for getting the daily activity summary.
- The *Unknown3* method was used for getting the data of the activity report.

Generic Data Acquisition Having recognized all the aforementioned API methods that are responsible for gathering medical data from the different activity trackers, the corresponding unified API was implemented based upon the data methods of *FIT9*, *FIT1*, and *ihealth1*, and finally collected the data from the Misfit activity tracker.

4.3 Discussion of Results

Through Table 5, it is clear that in order to identify and map ontologies, both syntactical and semantical mappings have to be applied. In more details, through Tables 2, 3, and 4 it can be seen that despite the fact that an ontology has been mapped with an ontology due to its syntactical similarity, the same ontology has been also mapped to a different ontology due to its semantical similarity, at the same time. It is clear that there are cases that an ontology has syntactical similarity with a specific API method (e.g., *Unknown3* has 53% syntactical match with the *FIT8* API method), but it does not have any semantic similarity (e.g., *Unknown3* has 52% semantical mapping with the *FIT4* API method). Consequently, we are not able to create patterns and rules mentioning that in the case that an ontology matches syntactically or semantically with a specific ontology, it has always an exact match with it. However, the overall mechanism provides reliable results, since all the provided results have been also calculated manually and compared with the aforementioned results.

5 Conclusions

It is an undeniable fact that mapping and identifying the different APIs and their methods in the IoT healthcare domain is far from solved. Currently, there exist a large number of attempts for covering most of the APIs' identification requirements through various techniques, based mainly on ontologies. However, none of these techniques promises the existence of a single global ontology any time soon, rising the needs of ontology mapping and semantics identification. For that reason, in this paper, we have studied the challenging topic of devices and data integration among heterogeneous medical devices for the IoT healthcare environments. We have considered data coming from different medical devices of both known and unknown API methods' nature, analyzing their APIs that are needed for the connection to these devices, and finally gathering data out of them.

Henceforth, a mechanism was proposed for effectively understanding the nature and the meaning of the different API methods that are being used by these medical devices, so as to collect their data through the corresponding API methods. In this mechanism, a global approach was proposed that had the ability to identify and construct ontologies of API methods of different medical devices, and then find the syntactic and semantic similarities between these ontologies. Through this way, the mechanism was able to understand the nature of the API methods that derive from these different medical devices, whose API methods' nature were primarily unknown. According to the results of the evaluation of the mechanism, it is not possible to create patterns or rules in order to understand the semantics of an ontology and match it with a different one, since there are cases that the syntactical or semantic similarity may produce results that overlap each other. However, this mechanism sounds promising since the derived results had exact match with the manual ontology mapping results that were calculated.

Nevertheless, writing an automated tool that would work between any ontologies is still a challenging task. In this context, we are working on the evaluation of the developed mechanism, by testing it with multiple heterogeneous medical devices. Our future work includes the development of a mechanism that will consider not only the devices' API methods URL paths and general descriptions, but also the format of the devices' sent data. Finally, we aim to extend our work by calculating through additional techniques the syntactic and the semantic similarities.

Acknowledgements The CrowdHEALTH project has received funding from the European Union's Horizon 2020 research and innovation programme under grant agreement No 727560.

References

1. Wang, W., et al.: A comprehensive ontology for knowledge representation in the internet of things. In: TrustCom, 2012 IEEE 11th International Conference on, pp. 1793–1798. IEEE (2012)
2. Global M2M market. https://machinaresearch.com/news/global-m2m-market-to-grow-to-27-billion-devices-generating-usd16-trillion-revenue-in-2024. Accessed 31 Oct 2018
3. How the next evolution of the internet is changing everything. https://www.cisco.com/c/dam/en/us/products/collateral/se/internet-of-things/at-a-glance-c45-731471.pdf. Accessed 31 Oct 2018
4. Jabbar, S., et al.: Semantic interoperability in heterogeneous IoT infrastructure for healthcare. Wirel. Commun. Mob. Comput. **2017**, 9731806 (2017)
5. Pham, C., et al.: Management architecture for heterogeneous IoT data sources in home network. In: Consumer Electronics, pp. 1–5. IEEE (2016)
6. Data integration and the healthcare industry. https://blogs.informatica.com/2016/06/09/data-integration-and-the-healthcare-industry/#fbid=OG3rCb7-tdh. Accessed 31 Oct 2018
7. Islam, S.R., et al.: The internet of things for health care: a comprehensive survey. IEEE Access. **3**, 678–708 (2015)
8. Kim, J., Lee, J.-W.: OpenIoT: an open service framework for the internet of things. In: Internet of Things, 2014 IEEE World Forum on, pp. 89–93. IEEE (2014)
9. Data integration in health care. http://link.springer.com/chapter/10.1007/978-3-319-56103-5_8. Accessed 31 Oct 2018
10. Gardner, S.P.: Ontologies and semantic data integration. Drug Discov. Today. **10**, 1001–1007 (2005)
11. Whose meaning? Which ontology? https://ontotext.com/meaning-ontology/. Accessed 31 Oct 2018
12. Buranarach, M., et al.: An Ontology-Based Framework for Development of Clinical Reminder System to Support Chronic Disease Healthcare. Ministry of Public Health, Nonthaburi (2009)
13. Noy, N. F., McGuinness, D. L.: Ontology development 101: a guide to creating your first ontology. SMI-2001-0880, Stanford Medical Informatics, Stanford (2001)

14. Calvanese, D., Giacomo, G.: Ontology-based data integration. In: Tutorial at the Semantic Days 2009 Conference Stavanger, Norway, 2009
15. Gagnon, M.: Ontology-based integration of data sources. In: Information Fusion, 10th International Conference on, pp. 1–8. IEEE (2007)
16. Spaccapietra, S., Parent, C.: View integration: a step forward in solving structural conflicts. IEEE Trans. Data Knowl. Eng. **6**(2), 258–274 (1994)
17. Ram, S., Park, J.: Semantic conflict resolution ontology (SCROL): an ontology for detecting and resolving data and schema-level semantic conflict. IEEE Trans. Knowl. Data Eng. **16**(2), 189–202 (2004)
18. Martín, L., et al.: Ontology Based Integration of Distributed and Heterogeneous Data Sources in ACGT, pp. 301–306. HEALTHINF, Setúbal (2008)
19. ACGT Project. http://acgt.ercim.eu/. Accessed 31 Oct 2018
20. Carbonaro, A., et al.: Integrating heterogeneous data of healthcare devices to enable domain data management. JeLKS. **14**(1), 1826-6223 (2018)
21. Pötter, B., Sztajnberg, A.: Adapting heterogeneous devices into an IoT context-aware infrastructure. In: Software Engineering for Adaptive and Self-Managing Systems, pp. 64–74. ACM, New York (2016)
22. OWL. https://www.w3.org/TR/owl-guide/. Accessed 31 Oct 2018
23. Globle, C., et al.: Transparent access to multiple bioinformatics information sources. IBM Syst. J. **40**(2), 534–551 (2001)
24. Donelson, L., et al.: The BioMediator system as a data integration tool to answer diverse biologic queries. Proc. Medinfo. **107**, 768–772 (2004)
25. Philippi, S.: Light-weight integration of molecular biological databases. Bioinformatics. **20**, 51–57 (2004)
26. Eckman, B., et al.: Optimized seamless integration of biomolecular data. In: IEEE Int. Conf. on Bioinformatics and Biomedical Engineering: 4–6 November 2001; Bethesda, Maryland, USA, pp. 23–32. IEEE Computer Society Press, Washington, DC (2001)
27. Gong, P.: Dynamic integration of biological data sources using the data concierge. Health Inf. Sci. Syst. **1**(1), 7 (2013)
28. Yachir, A., et al.: A comprehensive semantic model for smart object description and request resolution in the internet of things. Procedia Comput. Sci. **83**, 147–154 (2016)
29. Uzdanaviciute, V., Butleris, R.: Ontology-based foundations for data integration. In: 1st International Conference on Business Intelligence and Technology, pp. 34–39. IARIA, Wilmington (2011)
30. Zhang, L., et al.: An extended hybrid ontology approach to data integration. In: International Conference on Biomedical Engineering and Informatics, pp. 1–4. IEEE (2009)
31. Mavrogiorgou, A., et al.: Plug'n'play IoT devices: an approach for dynamic data acquisition from unknown heterogeneous devices. In: Conference on Complex, Intelligent, and Software Intensive Systems, pp. 885–895. Springer, Cham (2017)
32. Mavrogiorgou, A., et al.: A comparative study of classification techniques for managing IoT devices of common specifications. In: International Conference on the Economics of Grids, Clouds, Systems, and Services, pp. 67–77. Springer, Cham (2017)
33. WordNet. https://wordnet.princeton.edu/. Accessed 31 Oct 2018
34. Natural Language Process semantic analysis: definition. https://www.expertsystem.com/natural-language-process-semantic-analysis-definition/. Accessed 10 Oct 2018
35. What is an artificial neural network? https://www.digitaltrends.com/cool-tech/what-is-an-artificial-neural-network/. Accessed 31 Oct 2018
36. Svozil, D., et al.: Introduction to multi-layer feed-forward neural networks. Chemom. Intell. Lab. Syst. **39**(1), 43–62 (1997)
37. Schumann, J., Liu, Y.: Performance estimation of a neural network-based controller. In: International Symposium on Neural Networks, pp. 981–990. Springer, Berlin (2006)
38. Jiménez-Ruiz, E., et al.: Exploiting the UMLS metathesaurus in the ontology alignment evaluation initiative. In: E-LKR. CEUR-WS.org (2012)
39. NetBeans IDE. https://netbeans.org//. Accessed 31 Oct 2018

Part II
Security

Security Challenges and Suggested Solutions for e-Health Information in Modern Society

Nureni Ayofe Azeez and Charles Van der Vyver

1 Introduction

The evolution of Information and Communication Technology has influenced the traditional approach for healthcare practices in the world. This development is well noticed in a partial abandonment of paper-based medical prescription to electronic version particularly in most of the developed countries of the world [1]. The need to federate and integrate various electronic health information from various domains such as medical research laboratories, hospital, health insurance firms has led to the evolvement of a concept called electronic health (e-Health). Simply put, e-Health can simply be defined as the use of Information Technology (IT) infrastructure and e-commerce practices for processing, sharing, and manipulation of health information. It is however noted that different domains being involved in sharing of medical data have made the application very difficult to manage hence the need for cloud-based environment which allows collaborative sharing of information across multiple administrative domains [1]. Cloud computing has so many advantages among which is seamless transfer and sharing of medical information in a timely manner. It has also relieved healthcare providers the rigor involved in managing infrastructure and also provided them ample opportunity to familiarize with IT service providers [2]. It has been established in different academic papers that cloud computing offers numerous benefits ranging from scalability, cost effectiveness, agility enhancement of collaborative sharing of resources [3]. Despite its various advantages, there are security and privacy challenges that urgently deserve utmost attention for realization of its efficient and full-scale utilization [4]. Cryptographic

N. A. Azeez (✉) · C. Van der Vyver
School of Computer Science and Information Systems, North-West University, Vaal Triangle Campus, Vanderbijlpark, South Africa
e-mail: charles.vandervyver@nwu.ac.za

P. R. M. Inácio et al. (eds.), *5th EAI International Conference on IoT Technologies for HealthCare*, EAI/Springer Innovations in Communication and Computing,
https://doi.org/10.1007/978-3-030-30335-8_5

and non-cryptographic approaches have been used on several occasions to ensure preservation of security and privacy of health data in the cloud computing. Also, fine-grained as well as patient-centric access control schemes are commonly being used to achieve privacy in electronic health. In this paper, various security measures being used for protecting data are reviewed. Their strengths and weaknesses are also exposed. Effort was made to proffer better alternatives for securing e-Health data.

1.1 What is E-Health?

E-health is an emerging field in the intersection of medical informatics, public health, and business, referring to health services and information delivered or enhanced through the Internet and related technologies. In a broader sense, the term characterizes not only a technical development, but also a state-of-mind, a way of thinking, an attitude, and a commitment for networked, global thinking, to improve health care locally, regionally, and worldwide by using Information and Communication Technology [5].

1.2 Cloud-Based e-Health Models

Three types of cloud models are usually employed for rendering e-Health cloud services. They are private, public, and hybrid cloud.

Private Cloud

This model is considered the most secured of all the models. There is a complete restriction to the public internet. The Electronic Medical Records (EMRs) in a private cloud are only accessed by an authorized personnel of the healthcare institutions who are regarded to be trustworthy and reliable [6]. A private e-Health cloud is shown in Fig. 1.

Public Cloud

This model consists of a shared infrastructure that is in total control of the third-party provider. The services of this form of cloud system are procured from the Cloud Service Providers (CSPs). With this model, Electronic Health Records (EHRs) are usually shared among various organizations. The EHRs are very vulnerable to various attacks and manipulations because they are stored at off-premises servers that are under the control of CSPs. To circumvent this security challenge, efficient

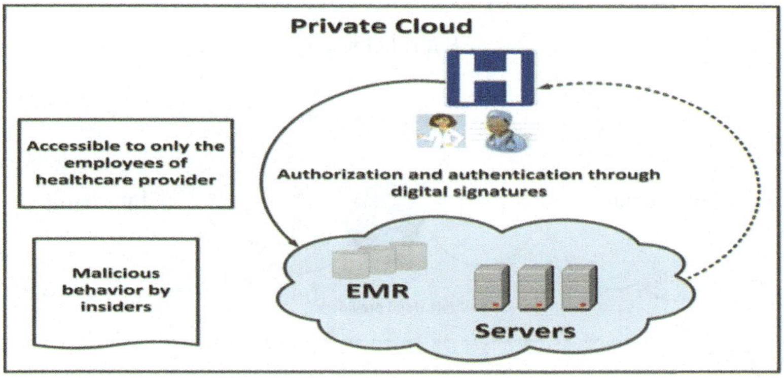

Fig. 1 An example of a private cloud in the context of e-Health [7]

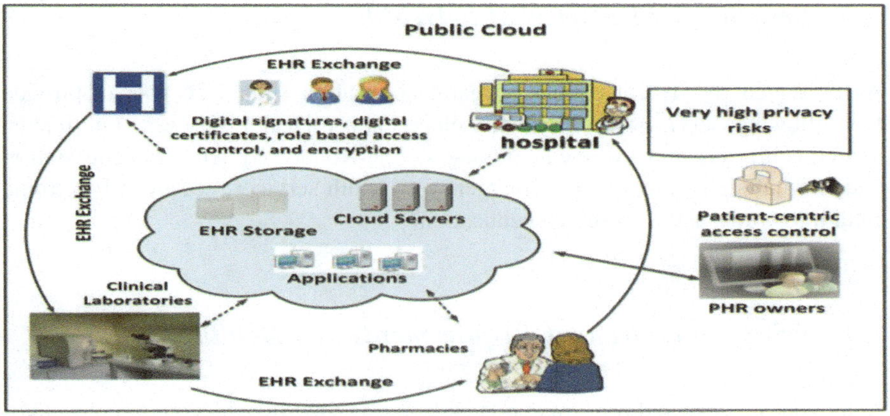

Fig. 2 An example of a public cloud in the context of e-Health [7]

cryptographic mechanisms and fine-grained access control frameworks are required [6]. An example of public cloud is depicted in Fig. 2.

Hybrid Cloud

This is a combination of both the private and public clouds such that each of the models operates individually but united through standard technologies [8]. The deployment of this model for e-Health is highly advantageous since it combines benefits of both models (public or private). Healthcare providers with restricted and limited physical resources as well as a strong interest in using legacy systems can conveniently make use of third-party services to house big medical data [9]. It however requires efficient security framework before it can be maximally utilized. An example of hybrid cloud is depicted in Fig. 3.

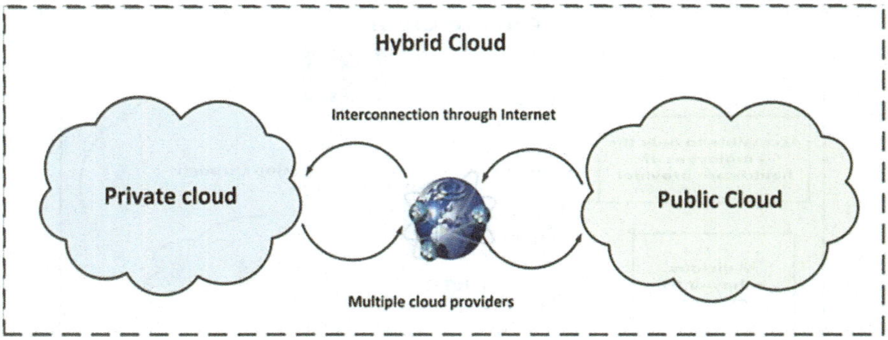

Fig. 3 An example of a hybrid cloud in the context of e-Health [7]

1.3 Benefits and Demerits of E-Health

As presented by [10], a typical e-Health application should be able to provide the following services: Findings for emergency e-Health services, multimedia conferencing, streaming of medical images, Tele-Robotic Systems, transmission of patient vital signs, findings for emergency e-Health services, access to Electronic Health Records, and research and education.

1.4 Privacy and Security Requirements in e-Health

Achieving security and privacy in e-Health is very vital in achieving the objectives of using this modern technology. This is very necessary as digitizing health-related data and sharing them may lead to different forms of attacks [11]. Many government health institutions have therefore developed framework to ensure high level of security and privacy. For instance, the Health Insurance Portability and Accountability Act (HIPAA) was put forward by the United States (US) Congress in 1996 as a federal law that applies to the US healthcare industry. In accordance with HIPAA [11] guidelines, a set of valuable security and privacy requirements must be put in place for effective utilization of e-Health. These are presented in Table 1.

2 Literature Review

This section presents a review of several articles in journals, conference proceedings, documents from the internet, book chapters, and books on various security approaches and mechanisms being used in e-Health. We did identify benefits and

Table 1 Security and privacy requirements as recommended by HIPAA

Requirement	Description
Patient's understanding	This implies that patients have an exclusive right to know and understand how their sensitive and private health information are kept and utilized by any healthcare provider
Patient's control	This allows patients to be given permission to determine who can access his/her health data
Confidentiality	Health information should be kept away from people who should not access it. The sanctity of the information should be maintained
Data integrity	This ensures that manipulation and omission of health information are totally prohibited. Hence, health information being shared should be a true representation of original information without any form of amendment or alteration
Consent exception	This stipulates that patient information could be accessed without his consent only in emergency cases
Non-repudiation	Healthcare practitioner should deny the fact that it has performed a certain activity on the sensitive data of patient. Such activity should be supported with evidence to avoid dispute or suspicion
Auditing	This is a requirement that health data should be well monitored frequently along with any form of activity to ensure that data is well secured and protected. This will assist user to know the confidential status of his data

demerits of each of the approaches. We also provided, in the next section, how those weaknesses could be taken care of.

Shin et al. [12] examined various security models for healthcare applications and attempted to see how information leakage could be protected. They evaluated various security requirements to ensure security and privacy in electronic health. To find solution to identified security challenges in electronic health, they employed extended RBAC security model. They came up with u-healthcare service integration platform where extended RBAC model was deployed.

The architecture was designed to carry out four main functions: exchanging health information, meal recommendation, transaction of health information, and management of health information on any smart devices [12]. It is however worthy of note that security issue was not properly resolved. The model is not suitable for a distributed environment. As a result, the solution provided has limited applications. The application does not also consider expansion in the number of users.

Simplicio et al. [13] present how a lightweight framework was used to present SecureHealth architecture that is based on Transport Layer Security/Secure Sockets Layer (TLS/SSL) for protecting data exchange with the server that requires no extra security layer. SecureHealth which includes many security features like authorization provides security services for transmitted and stored data. It has a good benefit of preventing alien from unauthorized access to the system that contains health information. Aside from this, it provides the manager the capability of identifying misnomer from information supplied [13]. Despite the benefits accrue from this framework, the main challenge is that it is platform dependent and not scalable. In a cloud-based environment, the security policy and framework must give room for scalability and future expansion.

In order to ensure that e-Health care service providers decrease the cost of maintaining data and allowing it to be available online in a secured manner, Barua et al. proposed a security mechanism with different levels of hierarchy. Provision of access control was carried out at a central level. They adopted Attribute Based Encryption (ABE) in such a way that privileges were mapped and juxtaposed into various roles with ABE access structures. The main challenge with this approach is the complexity of responding to various requests from different users due to storage of health information located in a centralized server [14]. Also, priority needs to be set when there is a simultaneous request by users.

In order to solve the challenge of having data storage of health information in a centralized server, Guo et al. [15] considered the distributed and collaborative nature of e-Health system. They did not allow a centralized server to handle authentication and authorization procedures, instead, they allowed both the patients and doctors to carry out authorization process. In fact, users are permitted to access based on their privileges without disclosing their attributes and identities. This framework addresses and solves the problem of handling and maintaining security, privacy as well as variability of all users attributes [15]. However, there is no room for collaborative sharing of medical data across different domains. The framework is too complex to implement. As of now, there is no real-life implementation to proof its efficiency as claimed by the authors.

Gajanayake et al. [16] came up with a special privacy and secured oriented access control architecture only for e-Health. They achieved their design by combining three different security models: Discretionary Access Control (DAC), Mandatory Access Control (MAC), and Role Based Access Control (RBAC) [17] to come up with a novel architecture which allows healthcare providers and patients to dictate and set access privileges. The major drawback of this framework is in its ability to be useful only as a standalone security model to attain health electronic record requirements [16].

A secured patient-centric electronic health information schema was proposed by Barua et al., for providing reliable access privilege in a cloud-based environment by using a protocol called Proxy Re-encryption. The schema which has five main stages makes use of Attribute Based Encryption to permit patient-centric access control. The performance analysis reveals that the schema has a good and excellent performance. The weakness is that it is not flexible enough for other forms of distributed systems. What is more, the schema does not give room for scalability and flexibility [14]. Only a limited number of users were considered during evaluation.

Kumar et al. [18] proposed a new framework for electronic health on encryption technique; Attribute Based Encryption (ABE) [19]. In this case, users are divided into two principal domains: personal and public domains. The essence of this is to handle key management complexity. In the personal domain, every owner is allowed to encrypt/access only data under his attributes, while the public domain allows users to adopt and make use of multi-authority ABE to enhance the security countermeasures [18]. The great challenge with this approach is the issue of scalability and flexibility because integrating Attribute Based Encryption into large scale Electronic Health Record system poses serious and great key management challenge.

Zhu et al. [20] proposed a secure and reliable framework that makes use of re-encryption and Attribute Based Encryption (ABE) with proxy encryption that is Rivest Shamir and Adleman (RSA) enabled. The objective of using proxy was to introduce separation mechanism to guarantee the validity of patient's data. In this case, only the professionals are given the write privilege keys, while the read privilege keys are given to patients [20]. The essence of this is to prevent full authorization by the patients. Through this framework, the computation overhead has been drastically reduced. With this approach, the healthcare practitioner can easily be prevented from getting the read keys without approval from both end. However, the scheme gives room for a limited number of users as it is not scalable.

Another secured model was proposed by Sunagar and Biradar. The secured framework is based on Advanced Encryption Standard (AES) algorithm developed to encrypt information about patients based on the security policy [21]. The security model allows users to maintain information in a reliable and secured manner in a cloud-based environment. The framework which has three modules guarantees high level of security and privacy. The drawback of this framework is that it could not work with all forms of operating systems. It is operating system dependent. It is also very complex to implement in a real-life scenario.

Liu et al. combined RBAC with Hierarchical Identity-Based Encryption (HIBE) schema to come up with an encryption technique for securing patient's data before they are outsourced to the storage data [22]. RBAC assists to facilitate user's privileges. The main weakness of this framework is that it does not provide reliable and accurate access control requirements. Patient may not access privileges to their confidential information without following HIPAA regulations.

Bahtiyar and Çağlayan proposed from the view point of an entity, a trust-based assessment security model for electronic health services [23]. The model which contains a detailed architecture that is applicable to various entities and servers as a unique trust assessment metrics may be used to evaluate a specific feature of a security system. The results obtained from simulation revealed that the framework gives better results in terms of trust computation when compared to the various existing trust models for e-health solutions. The model however is cumbersome, it contains some mathematical variables whose values were not clearly evaluated.

Shin et al. [12] evaluated various security requirements related to privacy in electronic healthcare services. They proposed an enhanced Role Based Access Control model to design u-healthcare service integration platform (u-HCSIP). The model which carries out four main functions is however unusable in a collaborative environment. It does not permit user to have exclusive privilege and dictate who should access his/her medical details [12]. The model is not implementable in a cloud-based environment.

The work of Li and Hoang centers on a novel role-interaction-organization privacy and security model with specific application to electronic health system and services [24]. The framework is modeled in the form of a multi-agent system. The role in the model determines both access privileges and initiates various requests to interact in a flexible manner with agents who satisfy the security requirements. To confirm the efficiency of the model, a simple case from electronic health system was used for performance evaluation. The main drawback with this model is that it is too generic. It also lacks security information aggregation.

The work of Fan et al. [25] also underscore the need for privacy in e-Health system. They carried out a design and implementation with the Single Point of Contact (SPoC) which guarantees claim-based authorization as well facilitates integration and deployment of reliable e-Health services to be hosted in a cloud-based domain [25]. The result of the model is fairly reliable. The application can only work with limited number of users. It is not flexible and dynamic enough for a very large number of users.

Bhartiya et al. [26] work on access control security model that uses a unique Hierarchy Similarity Analyzer (HSA). The model evaluates and assigns a Security_Level (SL) to users sharing data across different administrative domains. The SL ensures the approved and authorized percentage of data to be shared on any agreed collaboration of different policies. This security model allows combination of various policies and recognizes the likely policy-disparity culminating because of attribute conflicts in the set of defined rules [26]. The model was implemented using XACML policies and compared with other similar security models. One of the major challenges with this framework is in its inability to incorporate different types of policy-conflicts such as temporal constraints, semantic, and syntactic. Also, there is no absolute guarantee to security and privacy in any federated agencies [43].

Rezaeibagha and Mu [27] developed a novel access control framework to address the challenges of security and privacy in Electronic Health Record (EHR). The framework adopted hybrid clouds as well as access control policy transformation to guarantee reliable and dependable access control and authorization-preserving data sharing among different healthcare providers [27]. To make the model efficient, some cryptographic building blocks were introduced with access control policy transformation to tackle different users of EHR with different access privileges and permission in various cloud environments. The main drawback with this framework is its inability to give room for user's expansion. It does not give room for scalability because the number of users is limited [41].

In an attempt to find a solution to security issues in EHR, the duo of Garcia-Morchon and Wehrle developed a fine-grained access control for ubiquitous healthcare electronic applications. The framework enhances the existing traditional RBAC security model for two purposes. It explores it to allocate access policies to different sensor nodes and also stores very vital information such as health information, time, and location that are very critical to decision making on security [28]. The modular nature of the framework makes it easy and convenient for deployment of policies on various sensor networks. One of the main challenges of the model is lack of detection mechanism for illegal and unauthorized access in case of any emergency situation [42].

Efforts were made by Amini et al. [29], to come up with a lightweight security model for e-Health. In achieving this, they look into various set of security protocols like MiniSec, RC4-based as well as various ciphers algorithms such as RC4 and AES. The researchers applied the ciphers algorithms to combined attacks [29]. At the end of the experimentation, they confirmed that Skipjack cipher algorithms and RC4 are very efficient and reliable for achieving access confidentiality and integrity in Electronic Health. The authors fail however to investigate the efficient approaches for the remaining security requirements. Invariably, the conclusion drawn on the few algorithms investigated could not justify the conclusion that they are the best and most efficient.

Since it has been established that traditional Public Key Infrastructure (PKI) for implementing cryptographic mechanisms is cumbersome and time consuming, Wang et al. [30] described different related cryptographic techniques for ensuring security and privacy of Electronic Health system. They evaluated the performance analysis of these techniques which include Identity-Based Encryption (IBE) and new Identity-Based Proxy Re-encryption (IBPRE) Schemes [30]. From the evaluation, it was observed that newly developed IBPRE is better and efficient for re-encryption which can subsequently be used to protect health information in the cloud. The drawback with this technique is that the authors were unable to verify the performance of other encryption techniques, hence should not be categorical on the efficiency of the new IBPRE.

In a bid to secure medical data and other sensitive medical information, Karakış et al. [31] achieved this through the combination of medical data into one single file by using steganographic approach for hiding data. In their work, they proposed two new image steganography approaches that are dependent on fuzzy-logic and similarity. The objective of this was to allow for selection of the non-sequential least significant bits (LSB) of image pixels. They made use of the similarity values of the realized gray levels in the pixels hide the message [31]. With this approach, the message is protected to ward off any form of attack through lossless compression and symmetric encryption algorithms. The performance of steganographic image quality and rating was measured by Mean Square of Error (MSE), Peak Signal-to-Noise Ratio (PSNR), Structural Similarity Measure (SSIM), Universal Quality Index (UQI), and Correlation Coefficient (CC). With the results obtained, the newly proposed approach guarantees security and privacy of patient information and also increases data repository. The drawback of this approach is that it could not handle and tackle noise cancelation and data reduction which might enhance embedding capability.

After acknowledging the vulnerability nature of the cryptographic-based approaches for securing health records, Sahi et al. [32] did some technical review on some other security models being used to secure and protect electronic health information. They eventually proposed two main approaches to ensure security and privacy. The approaches are the Privacy-Preserving approach and the Security-Preserving approach on the one hand and a disaster recovery plan on the other hand [32]. The former approach is a robust mechanism for achieving both the privacy and integrity of medical information, while the latter approach could only be used for reliable and dependable authentication approach for electronic medical information. The main drawback is the inability of the mechanism to function efficiently if any of the approaches fails. The model is not also interoperable enough to be accommodated and implemented in a cloud-based environment.

Peleg et al. [33] critically studied RBAC and observed that it does not provide account for the reason under which request to access sensitive data is made. As a result of this weakness, they developed a framework with a Situation-Based Access Control (SitBAC) model. SitBAC is considered to be a conceptual framework that defines scenarios where a patient's access to electronic information is either denied or allowed [33]. SitBAC uses the Situation Schema which comprises of Patient's entities, Electronic Health Record (EHR), Data-Requestor along with their relations and properties. This model is considered to be generic which can also be used and adapted in other domains apart from medical information. One of the major weaknesses of this model is that it could not be able to factor in all the likely stakeholders with their various goals. Also, the model does not include a formal representation of the SitBAC as a knowledge base [39].

Rubio et al. [34] modified the security features in the Standard communications protocol for computer assisted electrocardiography (SCP-ECG) to allow file to be stored securely. The new security approach allows SCP-ECG files to be properly accessed (permitted or denied) to users for numerous reasons ranging from clinical teaching or research, interpretation of the test as well as consultation. Access privilege is supported by cryptographic elements that are well induced and scaled by means of role-based profiles [34]. The application has been confirmed to be very effective to authorize and authenticate users and protect the privacy of sensitive electronic health information. Despite the efficiency of the framework, the application cannot be deployed in a cloud based environment; hence, there is difficulty in using the model in a distributed environment. The model is technical and difficult to implement. There is no real-life implementation to justify its efficiency and capability [40].

Adoption of two-stage key access control and zero-knowledge protocol was considered by [35] for e-Health system. In order to obtain a secure connection between various entities DUKPT and a two-stage combination of key encryption were adopted. The framework was analyzed with respect to resistance to common attacks and data confidentiality. The proposed scheme tolerates a good number of simultaneous authorization requests with excellent response time. The main drawback with this scheme is that it has limited number of entities: users U, a cloud server CS, a service provider SP, and an authentication and access control manager AAM. This implies that it is not scalable; this is not good for a cloud-based environment because it will not give room for collaborative sharing of resources.

Another framework for access control to Personal Health Records (PHRs) in a distributed environment was proposed by [36]. They leveraged Attribute Based Encryption (ABE) security model to encrypt patients' data in order to attain and achieve scalable access control as well as fine-grained access for PHRs. The system was divided into multiple security domains in order to reduce the complexity that may arise due to key distribution. In this case, each domain manages only a small percentage of the users. Users are given absolute control over their own privacy. The scheme is dynamic in nature as it supports on-demand withdrawal of user's access privileges. The scheme however fails to support more expressive owner-defined access control policies.

A novel patient-centric scheme with good framework for data access control to electronic health records was proposed by [4]. They identified scalability and fine-grained access as part of the challenges. They therefore optimized and leveraged Attribute Based Encryption (ABE) models to secure and encrypt patient's PHR data. They focused on a situation where there is multiple data ownership and divide the user into various security domains. This was done to reduce the key management complexity for both the owners and users. With the exploitation of multi-authority ABE there is a better performance of patience privacy and security. The scheme allows flexible modification of various file attributes. Despite the claims by the authors, the proposed framework was only simulated and it has not been tested on a real-life case to establish the claim. The results obtained could not guarantee efficiency of the framework when tested in a real-life situation. Also, few users were also considered. The authors failed to inform what may happen when there is increase in the number of entities [38].

3 Future Directions on Security of e-Health

It has been established that remarkable progress has been made regarding security and privacy in e-Health in cloud-based environment. It is also very significant to suggest few approaches to ensure and enforce security measures in e-Health system. Doing this is aimed at maintaining and enhancing efficiency of the security and privacy initiatives. Hence the followings strategies are proposed as the new security solutions:

(a) We are of the opinion that auditing will assist at ensuring security and privacy in e-Health. It will assist in locating and identifying any form of misconduct that could affect e-Health solution. Hence, auditing should be considered as a new research direction for e-Health solution;
(b) From the available and reviewed literatures, we discovered that most e-Health solutions use encryption scheme to ensure and achieve security and privacy. We are of the opinion that encrypting the parts or sections which reveal the information about the e-Health user will be excellent as the remaining part of the data is left unencrypted. Doing this will not in any way lead to insecurity of data;
(c) Most solutions utilized RBAC model to ensure security and privacy in e-Health. We are of the view that Attribute Based Access Control (ABAC) model should be used to ensure excellent scalability and flexibility for authentications and authorizations;
(d) Attribute Based Encryption (ABE) is known to be excellent in ensuring privacy in e-Health, but excessive computations while decrypting data are imminent and affect its performance because of bilinear pairing operations. We are also

of the opinion that finding solution to this bilinear operations will enhance the efficiency of ABE. Searching for the solution is considered a good research area for e-Health;

(e) General enforcement of privacy requirements should be adopted. Most of the solutions focused mainly on the security and privacy of patients. Privacy of all parties involved in electronic health systems should be incorporated. Getting the required security and privacy violations will be a good research area;

(f) Based on the literatures reviewed, it was noted that some solutions adopted RBAC, MAC, and DAC. We are of the opinion that these models will perform better if they are hybridized to form a single model for ensuring security and privacy in e-Health. This is a very good and interesting area of research which researchers could focus on in e-Health.

4 Features of the Proposed System

The motive behind this architecture is to build a secured, dynamic, and dependable framework for E-Health. The architectural framework is to be absolutely controlled by the patient who is considered a major stakeholder in E-health system.

A patient will obtain his full access through authentication into a designated medical institution (hospital). At this point, he chooses who his medical personnel is. A medical officer (MO) will have access to patient's information that is available in the cloud by using Access Control List (ACL) security model [37]. The type of activity to carry out on a patient will be regulated by Mandatory Access Control (MAC) [37] security model.

Mandatory Access Control (MAC) is a type of security model that permits operating system to coerce the ability of an initiator of an action to carry out some operations on a target or an object. An object is regarded as constructs such as files, IO devices, or memory segments, while a subject could be regarded as a thread or a process.

Access Control List (ACL) on the other hand is a security model that provides a set of permission attached to objects. It indicates who among the users or processes should be granted access privilege to objects. It also specifies what operations are permitted on given objects [37].

The architecture permits proxy to give room for quick attendance to any patience in case of an emergency.

Figure 4 shows the proposed architecture for privacy in e-health. The performance of the architecture is expected to provide high degree of reliability, dependability, and efficiency in protecting patient information after its full implementation. Specifically, the architecture is expected to give room for flexible authentication to e-Health information on patient. Also, it is expected to give absolute control (either directly or through proxy) of information by the major stakeholders as well as providing mechanism for emergency and complex situations whenever the need arises.

Procedure 1. Step for dynamic patient-regulated access framework
1. A patient seeks medical consultation
2. Patient uses authentication to gain admission to the hospital using his ID/proxy (proxy isrequired in case of emergency)
3. Application of access control list (ACL) in the selection of a doctor to access patient'sinformation from electronic health server (EHR)
4. Access by a doctor into the cloud is regulated by mandatory access control (MAC) on thenature of activities to be carried out
5. There is a doctor–patient feedback server that provides feedback on patient via the doctor'sreport
6. Report obtained in (v) will be accessed through authorization by the patient
7. Patient takes the result to pharmacy department for drug collection

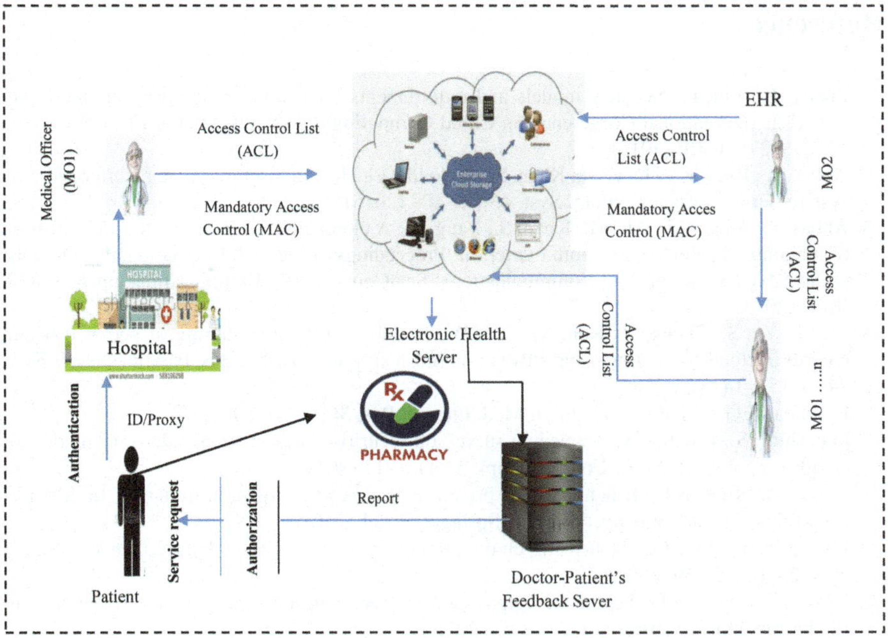

Fig. 4 Proposed security architecture for electronic health

5 Conclusion

It is very vital to implement e-Health solution in any country of the world to enhance excellent healthcare delivery system. To maximally enjoy the services of e-Health, it is very important and fundamental to put in place the required security and privacy mechanisms to prevent any form of security breach and vulnerability. From the foregoing, we have been able to review literatures on security and privacy in e-Health and also identified lapses in the existing solutions. In order to have an efficient e-Health solution, it is important we incorporate some of the suggested solutions proposed in any model being proposed for e-Health solution. The government and policymakers in all countries of the world should develop a comprehensive e-Health document framework to motivate and enable its acceptance. Governments should also develop research institutes where security experts will come together to brainstorm on how to develop e-Health solution that would be secured enough from any form of vulnerability. There should be detailed privacy regulations on the services and practices of e-Health so that patients can feel highly protected while disclosing their health-related information. Finally, we proposed a secured architecture for electronic health that could guarantee efficiency, reliability, and regulated access framework to health information.

References

1. Zhang, R., Liu, L.: Security models and requirements for healthcare application clouds. In: 3rd IEEE International Conference on Cloud Computing (CLOUD), Miami, FL, USA, USA, pp. 268–275. IEEE (2010)
2. Abbas, A., Bilal, K., Zhang, L., Khan, S.: A cloud based health insurance plan recommendation system. Future Gener. Comput. Syst. **43**, 99–109 (2015)
3. Abbas, A., Khan, M., Ali, M., Khan, S., Yang, L.: A cloud based framework for identification of influential health experts from twitter. In: Proceedings of the 15th International Conference on Scalable Computing and Communications (ScalCom) (2015), Beijing, China, pp. 831–838. IEEE (2015)
4. Li, M., Yu, S., Zheng, Y., Ren, K., Lou, W.: Scalable and secure sharing of personal health records in cloud computing using attribute-based encryption. IEEE Trans. Parallel Distrib. Syst. **24**(1), 131–143 (2012)
5. Eysenbach, G.: What is e-health? J. Med. Internet Res. **3**(2), e20 (2001)
6. Subashini, S., Kavitha, V.: Review: a survey on security issues in service delivery models of cloud computing. J. Netw. Comput. Appl. **34**(1), 1–11 (2011)
7. Abbas, A., Khan, S.U.: E-health cloud: privacy concerns and mitigation strategies. In: Medical Data Privacy Handbook, pp. 389–421. Springer, Basel (2015)
8. Zissis, D., Lekkas, D.: Addressing cloud computing security issues. Future Gener. Comput. Syst. **28**(3), 583–592 (2012)
9. VMware: Your cloud in healthcare. http://www.vmware.com/files/pdf/VMware-Your-Cloudin-Healthcare-Industry-Brief.pdf. Accessed 2015
10. Skorin-Kapov, L., Matijasevic, M.: Analysis of QoS requirements for e-health services and mapping to evolved packet system QoS classes. Int. J. Telemed. Appl. **2010**, 1–19 (2010)
11. Pussewalage, H., Oleshchuk, V.: Privacy preserving mechanisms for enforcing security and privacy requirements in E-health solutions. Int. J. Inf. Manag. **36**(6), 1161–1173 (2016)
12. Shin, M., Jeon, H., Ju, Y., Lee, B., Jeong, S.: Constructing RBAC based security model in u-healthcare service platform. Sci. World J. **2015**, 937914 (2015)
13. Simplicio, M., Iwaya, L., Barros, B., Carvalho, T., Naslund, M.: SecourHealth: a delay-tolerant security framework for mobile health data collection. IEEE J. Biomed. Health Inform. **19**(2), 761–772 (2015)
14. Barua, M., Lu, R., Liang, X., Shen, X.: PEACE: an efficient and secure patient-centric access control scheme for eHealth care system. In: The First International Workshop on Security in Computers, Networking and Communications, Shanghai, China, pp. 970–975. IEEE (2011)
15. Guo, L., Zhang, C., Sun, J., Fang, Y.: PAAS: a privacy-preserving attribute-based authentication system for eHealth networks. In: 2012 32nd IEEE International Conference on Distributed Computing Systems, Macau, China, pp. 224–233. IEEE (2012)

16. Gajanayake, R., Iannella, R., Sahama, T.: Privacy oriented access control for electronic health records. e-J. Health Inform. **8**(2), 175–186 (2014)
17. Azeez, N., Ademolu, O.: CyberProtector: identifying compromised URLs in electronic mails with Bayesian classification. In: International Conference Computational Science and Computational Intelligence (CSCI), Las Vegas, NV, USA, pp. 959–965. IEEE (2016)
18. Kumar, M., Fathima, M., Mahendran, M.: Personal health data storage protection on cloud using MA-ABE. Int. J. Comput. Appl. **75**(8), 11–16 (2013)
19. Ayofe, A.N., Adebayo, S.B., Ajetola, A.R., Abdulwahab, A.F.: A framework for computer aided investigation of ATM fraud in Nigeria. Int. J. Soft Comput. **5**(3), 78–82 (2010)
20. Zhu, H., Huang, R., Liu, X., Li, H.: SPEMR: a new secure personal electronic medical record scheme with privilege separation. In: 2014 IEEE International Conference on Communications Workshops (ICC), Sydney, NSW, Australia, pp. 700–705. IEEE (2014)
21. Sunagar, V., Biradar, C.: Securing public health records in cloud computing patient centric and fine grained data access control in multi owner settings. Int. J. Sci. Appl. Inf. Technol. **3**(4), 18–21 (2014)
22. Liu, W., Liu, X., Liu, J., Wu, Q., Zhang, J., Li, Y.: Auditing and revocation enabled role-based access control over outsourced private EHRs. In: 2015 IEEE 17th International Conference on High Performance Computing and Communications (HPCC), New York, NY, USA, pp. 336–341. IEEE (2015)
23. Bahtiyar, S., Çağlayan, M.: Trust assessment of security for e-health systems. Electron. Commer. Res. Appl. **13**(3), 164–177 (2014)
24. Li, W., Hoang, D.: A new security scheme for e-health system. In: International Symposium on Collaborative Technologies and Systems, 2009. CTS '09., Baltimore, MD, USA, pp. 361–366. IEEE (2009)
25. Fan, L., Lo, O., Buchanan, W., Ekonomou, E., Sharif, T., Sheridan, C.: SPoC: protecting patient privacy for e-health services in the cloud. In: eTELEMED 2012, pp. 1–6. IARIA, Wilmington (2014)
26. Bhartiya, S., Mehrotra, D., Girdhar, A.: Proposing hierarchy-similarity based access control framework: a multilevel electronic health record data sharing approach for interoperable environment. J. King Saud Univ. Comput. Inf. Sci. **29**(4), 505–519 (2017)
27. Rezaeibagha, F., Mu, Y.: Distributed clinical data sharing via dynamic access-control policy transformation. Int. J. Med. Inform. **89**, 25–31 (2016)
28. Garcia-Morchon, O., Wehrle, K.: Efficient and context-aware access control for pervasive medical sensor networks. In: 2010 8th IEEE International Conference on Pervasive Computing and Communications Workshops (PERCOM Workshops), Mannheim, Germany, pp. 322–327. IEEE (2010)
29. Amini, S., Verhoeven, R., Lukkien, J., Chen, S.: Toward a security model for a body sensor platform. In: 2011 IEEE International Conference on Consumer Electronics (ICCE), Las Vegas, NV, USA, pp. 143–144. IEEE (2011)
30. Wang, X., Ma, J., Xhafa, F., Zhang, M., Luo, X.: Cost-effective secure E-health cloud system using identity based cryptographic techniques. Futur. Gener. Comput. Syst. **67**, 242–254 (2017)
31. Karakış, R., Güler, I., Çapraz, I., Bilir, E.: A novel fuzzy logic-based image steganography method to ensure medical data security. Comput. Biol. Med. **67**, 172–183 (2015)
32. Sahi, A., Lai, D., Li, Y.: Security and privacy preserving approaches in the eHealth clouds with disaster recovery plan. Comput. Biol. Med. **78**, 1–8 (2016)
33. Peleg, M., Beimel, D., Dori, D., Denekamp, Y.: Situation-based access control: privacy management via modeling of patient data access scenarios. J. Biomed. Inform. **41**, 1028–1040 (2008)
34. Rubio, O., Alesanco, A., García, J.: A robust and simple security extension for the medical standard SCP-ECG. J. Biomed. Inform. **46**(1), 142–151 (2013)
35. Azeez, N.A., Lasisi, A.A.: Empirical and statistical evaluation of the effectiveness of four lossless data compression algorithms. Niger. J. Technol. Dev. **13**(2), 64–73 (2016)

36. Nureni, A.A., Irwin, B.: Cyber security: challenges and the way forward. Comput. Sci. Telecommun. **29**, 56–69 (2010)
37. Azeez, N., Venter, I.: Towards ensuring scalability, interoperability and efficient access control in a multi-domain grid-based environment. SAIEE Afr. Res. J. **104**(2), 54–68 (2013)
38. Kahani, N., Elgazzar, K., Cordy, K.: Authentication and access control in e-health systems in the cloud. In: IEEE International Conference on High Performance and Smart Computing (HPSC), Big Data Security on Cloud (BigDataSecurity), New York, NY, USA, pp. 13–23. IEEE (2016)
39. Li, M., Yu, S., Ren, K., Lou, W.: Securing personal health records in cloud computing: patient-centric and fine-grained data access control in multi-owner settings. In: International Conference on Security and Privacy in Communication Systems, pp. 89–106. Springer, Berlin (2010)
40. Azeez, N.A., Olayinka, A.F., Fasina, E.P., Venter, I.M.: Evaluation of a flexible column-based access control security model for medical-based information. J. Comput. Sci. Appl. **22**(1), 14–25 (2015)
41. Azeez, N.A., Babatope, A.B.: AANtID: an alternative approach to network intrusion detection. J. Comput. Sci. Appl. **23**(1), 129–143 (2016)
42. Azeez, N.A., Iliyas, H.D.: Implementation of a 4-tier cloud-based architecture for collaborative health care delivery. Niger. J. Technol. Dev. **13**(1), 17–25 (2016)
43. Azeez, N.A., Iyamu, T., Venter, I.M.: Grid security loopholes with proposed countermeasures. In: Gelenbe, E., Lent, R., Sakellari, G. (eds.) 26th International Symposium on Computer and Information Sciences, pp. 411–418. Springer, London (2011)

Part III
Monitoring and Rehabilitation

Telemonitoring Devices and Systems: Current Status and Future Trends

Liliana Tavares Machadeiro, Pedro Dinis Gaspar, and Miguel Castelo-Branco

1 Introduction

The number of individuals suffering from one of the various chronic diseases, which according to the World Health Organization (WHO) may also be referred to as no communicable diseases, has been increasing [1]. The significant increase in the average life expectancy at birth in recent years is an important and contributory factor, resulting in a greater focus on the disease in the elderly, who in future will be the large part of the population. These diseases are largely responsible for the expense of national health systems, which nowadays face major problems with scarce financial and human resources. From the point of view of the chronic patient, the expenses with the disease are high due to the medication costs and continuous monitoring and support that the disease demands [2]. Chronic patients are considered the main responsible for the increasing use of medical, hospital and emergency services. Thus, a special care that considers monitoring certain physical and biological parameters associated with the disease is required [3].

So, the need to find solutions to provide healthcare where good management of chronic diseases is performed, addressing the problem of the shortage of health

L. T. Machadeiro
University of Beira Interior, Covilhã, Portugal

P. D. Gaspar (✉)
University of Beira Interior, Covilhã, Portugal

C-MAST - Centre for Mechanical and Aerospace Science and Technologies,
University of Beira Interior, Covilhã, Portugal
e-mail: dinis@ubi.pt

M. Castelo-Branco
University of Beira Interior, Covilhã, Portugal

CICS-UBI – Health Sciences Research Centre, University of Beira Interior, Covilhã, Portugal

P. R. M. Inácio et al. (eds.), *5th EAI International Conference on IoT Technologies for HealthCare*, EAI/Springer Innovations in Communication and Computing,
https://doi.org/10.1007/978-3-030-30335-8_6

professionals by effectively allocating the available resources [4], is growing and it is believed that passes through telehealth devices and/or systems [5]. Telehealth, e-health, m-health and telemonitoring are quickly evolving and are already part of health systems. However, in the future, telemonitoring may become critical in the treatment of chronic diseases [3].

Telemonitoring consists in accomplishing the distant monitoring of patients, i.e., monitoring them remotely from the comfort of their home or beyond it [6]. Thus, there is an automonitoring of biological and physical parameters of the patient outside the hospital environment performed by itself or by a health provider, and the data is transmitted to the health care systems using information and communications technology (ICT).

The use of telemonitoring devices and systems can provide a safe and effective monitoring of these patients. The measurement of physical and biological parameters essential for the analysis of the evolution and treatment of the disease prescribed by the health professionals allows them to evaluate the data and take decisions to change or maintain prescriptions or health care for the monitored patient [4, 7].

Telemonitoring combines several advantages for patients with chronic diseases as well as for health systems. For the patient, telemonitoring allows the promotion of a better self-control that results in a better quality of life [2]. In the background, it allows the early detection of warning signs that consequently decrease the hospitalizations of these patients [4]. For the healthcare systems, the lack of health professionals and the lack of financial resources can be diminished by telemonitoring these patients. Health institutions will in future experience difficulties in caring for patients and their hospitalization. The growing number of patients is related also to the increasing trend of average life hope [4].

It is perceived that there is a problem in the health systems that will follow a worldwide worsening trend in the near future. The part of this problem can be surpassed with the growth of telemonitoring in the health sector, and particularly fostering the telemonitoring physical and/or biological parameters of patients with different chronic diseases.

This paper describes the evaluation carried out concerning the current status of telemonitoring devices and systems existing in the market and in some cases in the development phase. Their technical specifications, characteristics and their advantages for patients and health systems are described. In addition, the future trend for the development of this type of devices and system is analysed. Proposals for the implementation of new telemonitoring devices and systems for the support and management of chronic diseases are performed.

2 Methods

It is essential to introduce telemonitoring devices and systems into the daily life of chronically ill patients. As this condition is becoming a reality, a research and a description of some of market-available telemonitoring devices and systems applied to different chronic pathologies is performed. The selection of chronic diseases described within the paper was performed according to two criteria: (1) prevalence of chronic diseases, and preference was given to those with the highest incidence in the population; (2) frequency of information found in academic and scientific databases, such as PubMed, IEEE and B-on. Additionally, the technical specifications were gathered from the web pages of companies manufacturing or distributing telemonitoring devices and systems referenced in reports prepared by the Market Reports Center.

Proposals are performed to improve the technical specifications of the future telemonitoring devices and/or systems based on the ones existing in the market.

3 State of the Art on IoT Telemonitoring Medical Devices

The telemonitoring devices and systems discussed in this article were HealthGO Mini, VITALS360®, CareHomePod and HomePod, iSpO2®, EQ Connect™, eNephro, Prototype Device, eCareCompanion, Genesis Telemonitor, Honeywell HomMed, TCare Cardio Monitor and Smartheart™. These telemonitoring devices and systems are applied to chronic diseases such as Diabetes mellitus, Chronic Obstructive Pulmonary Disease (COPD) and Asthma, Chronic Kidney Disease, Thromboembolic Diseases and Heart Failure.

3.1 Telemonitoring Devices Used in Diabetes Mellitus

Diabetes mellitus is characterized as being a metabolic disease in which there is hyperglycaemia resulting from defective insulin secretion, insulin action or both. Chronic hyperglycaemia of diabetes is associated with long-term damage, such as dysfunction and failure of various organs, especially eyes, kidneys and heart [8]. According to the International Diabetes Federation (IDF) in 2011, 35 million adults had Type 1 or Type 2 diabetes. The estimate for 2030 is that there are 43 million adults with diabetes [9].

Diabetes management in Europe alone entails huge costs for health systems. In 2011, 89 million euros were spent on the treatment of diabetes and its complications, with no indirect costs being accounted for, which can increase the associated costs dramatically [9]. In the year 2013, IDF accounted for about 206 million diagnosed diabetics globally. The costs associated with Type 2 diabetic patients alone are about two to three times higher compared to a person of the same sex and the same age without the disease. Approximately 80% of the costs that this disease brings to health systems are the treatment of complications resulting from poor management of the disease [10].

According to IDF, the costs associated with diabetes will increase greatly due not only to the expected increase in the number of patients but also to the associated costs due to complications caused by poor management of the disease [9].

Monitoring glycaemic control in diabetic patients is essential. This procedure, repeated throughout the day along with taking the correct medication is essential to avoid complications of the disease. These patients have direct contact with the specialty doctor on average every 3 months or every 4 months, where adjustments are made to the therapy. In the intervals of these consultations, the dosages of medication may have to be changed to an efficacy of disease management. This is made difficult by the fact that the patient does not have the medical advice to do so [10].

Following is a set of commercially available diabetes mellitus telemonitoring devices. The devices described are HealthGO Mini, VITALS360® and Care-HomePod and HomePod. The CareHomePod is used in multi-resident homes and the HomePod is used in singular-resident homes. All devices have the portable advantage, allowing patients to take them in the event of a need to travel. The HealthGO Mini and CareHomePod and HomePod work as platforms that receive data collected by other devices, in this case, the blood glucose metre that diabetic patients use to obtain the blood glucose value that they connect with the platform (HealthGO Mini) via Bluetooth or USB and with the tablet (CareHomePod and HomePod) via Bluetooth. In the case of the VITALS360® device, it already has a built-in blood glucose metre that allows the blood glucose test to be performed directly on the device [11–13].

The process of obtaining the glycaemic value is invasive in all devices and platforms; being through the puncture to obtain a drop of blood that is placed on a test tape that is previously placed in the blood glucose metre. After this process, the glycaemic values obtained are sent through Wi-Fi to databases of each device that allow the analysis of these data by specialized health professionals who subsequently make the decision how to act. The device-to-patient interface is simple on all devices but customizable to the patient only VITALS360® and CareHomePod and HomePod have this feature [11, 13, 14]. Table 1 compares the technical specifications of telemonitoring devices and systems found for Diabetes mellitus disease.

Table 1 Comparison of technical specifications of telemonitoring devices used in Diabetes mellitus

	Device 1	Device 2	Device 3
Designation	HealthGO Mini	VITALS360®	CareHomePod; HomePod
Portability	Yes	Yes	Yes
Invasiveness	Yes	Yes	Yes
Interface	Not customized and simple	Custom and simple	Custom and simple
Connectivity	BluetoothUSBWi-Fi	Wi-Fi	BluetoothWi-Fi
Interoperability	No	No	No

It is concluded that all the described devices present very similar technical specifications, being overall only distinguished by the functionalities related to the connectivity, which are fundamental for any telemonitoring device, as well as for the man–machine interface. Interoperability is the missing technical specification in the three telemonitoring devices and systems analysed. However, as long as there is no international regulation that mandates and imposes manufacturers to provide this functionality in their devices, all will continue to use closed proprietary systems. It is important to remember that interoperability between systems and devices will have to be followed by strict legal and regulatory policies and standards related to data encryption to ensure their confidentiality. Some steps are taken in this direction by the Food and Drug Administration (FDA) in the United States of America (USA) as well as the European Commission (EC) in the European Union (EU).

3.2 Telemonitoring Devices Used in COPD and Asthma

Chronic Obstructive Pulmonary Disease (COPD) is a very common disease and is characterized by a progressive decrease in lung capacity and acute respiratory exacerbations [15]. In COPD there is a limitation of progressive respiratory flow, which may be partially or totally irreversible, associated with a chronic inflammatory response that increases harmful particles or gases in the airways and lungs [16]. In this disease, the loss of respiratory muscle function and airway obstruction is progressive [16], resulting in frequent hospital admissions, incapacity for the patient with this disease and also depression [17].

These patients suffer with the gradual worsening of some symptoms and also of lung function for a few days, such as exacerbations, sinus tachycardia, dyspnoea and hypoxemia. The early recognition by patients of these serious symptoms is not always achieved in order to avoid hospitalization. These symptomatologic events contribute significantly to a worsening of the disease, by deteriorating the respiratory health of the patient, and consequently also contribute to a lower quality of life for the patient [15, 16].

It is estimated that by 2020 the costs associated with the disease in the USA reach $49 billion annually. These costs are mostly due to hospital admissions due to exacerbations [18].

Asthma, which can be referred to as a form of COPD, is a disease that presents problems on a global scale and affects both the quality of life of patients who are carriers, as well as health systems because it is a high cost disease [19]. This disease is one of the most frequent chronic diseases and has been increasing its frequency in the last decade [20]. Only in the EU and the USA it affects about 5–6% of the population. Asthma and other forms of COPD require management, self-management and monitoring in order to control the symptoms of the disease with therapies adjusted to the condition of each patient and also to reduce the risk of exacerbations [16, 20]. The vast majority of asthmatic patients undergo corticosteroid therapy by inhalation and with drugs called β-adrenergic agonists, and a proportion of these patients require additional drugs such as oral corticosteroids [20].

Some biological parameters are important both for the diagnosis of the disease, as well as for its monitoring in the hospital environment and daily in the home. Pulmonary function is a biological parameter that fits perfectly into this definition [19].

The devices analysed are CareHomePod and HomePod, VITALS360® and iSpO2®. All devices have the portability characteristic, enabling patients to use them in the event of a need to travel. The iSpO2® is an adaptive device for an android smartphone or iOS, which functions as a pulse oximeter [21]. In the case of CareHomePod and HomePod the oximeter sends the values collected for these devices through Bluetooth and the VITALS360® has a built-in oximeter. Again, the processes of obtaining the values is not invasive in all devices and platforms. Then, measured values are sent through Wi-Fi to databases. The data is analysed by specialized health professionals who subsequently decide how to act. The interface of the device to the patient is simple on all devices and customizable to the patient [12, 21].

Table 2 reviews the technical specifications of the devices and telemonitoring systems found for COPD and Asthma.

The comparative results present the same conclusions as in the case of diabetes mellitus. Interoperability is the missing technical specification in the three devices and systems of telemonitoring analysed.

3.3 *Telemonitoring Systems Used in Chronic Kidney Disease*

Chronic kidney disease is a progressive disease that irreversibly impairs kidney structure and function [22].

Table 2 Comparison of technical specifications of telemonitoring devices used in DPOC and Asthma

	Device 1	Device 2	Device 3
Designation	CareHomePod; HomePod	VITALS360®	iSpO2®
Portability	Yes	Yes	Yes
Invasiveness	No	No	No
Interface	Custom and simple	Custom and simple	Custom and simple
Connectivity	Bluetooth Wi-Fi	Wi-Fi	Direct connection to smartphone Wi-Fi
Interoperability	No	No	No

Chronic kidney disease is associated with high morbidity, mortality and also high health expenditure. Factors such as diabetes mellitus, hypertension and cardiovascular diseases may contribute to the onset of chronic kidney disease. Thus, the prevalence of chronic kidney disease is increasing globally [23]. In the USA in 2006, the prevalence of chronic kidney disease in the adult population over 65 years of age at stage 3 was estimated to be 7.6 million patients at stage 4 of 400,000 patients and at stage 5 of 300,000 patients [24].

Chronic kidney patients in the early stages of the disease may be asymptomatic, leading to a lack of demand for medical care. Timely care of these patients can lead to a reduction in morbidity, mortality, costs associated with the disease, as well as a reduction in the number of consultations required for the patient, as the responsiveness of health systems tends to decrease [25, 26].

The economic burden on health systems increases as the disease progresses, with the greatest burden being on the last stage involving dialysis, hemodialysis or renal transplantation. Avoiding reaching these stages is important. Controlling the disease is fundamental, preventing its progression and consequently alleviating the economic burden, minimizing hospitalizations and improving the patient's quality of life [27].

In some situations not reaching the last stage of the disease becomes impossible. Peritoneal dialysis becomes the best solution for these patients. Telemonitoring combined with dialysis becomes a fundamental point, thus increasing the bet in this area [28].

In order to provide optimal care for these patients, telemonitoring becomes an essential component of health systems in the care of chronic kidney patients [25]. Telemonitoring combined with self-monitoring in these patients is essential in preventing disease progression and consequently in reducing hospitalizations [26].

Many telemonitoring systems applied to chronic kidney disease are still under development. In the following description of the devices, only the first device is already on the market. With all the rest only case studies were done to see if they are effective in the disease, having all had great success with proven effectiveness. The systems described are EQ Connect™, eNephro and Prototype Device. All systems present the portable advantage, enabling patients to use them aboard. This feature is largely due to the fact that they are web and android applications that receive the specific disease-related data predefined by specialized healthcare professionals through the manual introduction of data by the patient. The measuring process is non-invasive. The results are sent through Wi-Fi to databases to be analysed by specialized health professionals. The device interface to the patient is simple and customizable to the patient in the EQ Connect™ and eNephro application. The Prototype Device (still in development) is not customizable to the patient [24, 26, 29].

Table 3 reviews the technical specifications of telemonitoring systems found for Chronic Kidney Disease. Again, the results are similar. Interoperability is the missing technical specification in the three telemonitoring systems analysed.

Table 3 Comparison of technical specifications of telemonitoring systems used in Chronic Kidney Disease

	Device 1	Device 2	Device 3
Designation	EQ Connect™	eNephro	Prototype device
Portability	Yes	Yes	Yes
Invasiveness	No	No	No
Interface	Custom and simple	Custom and simple	Not customized and simple
Connectivity	Wi-Fi	Wi-Fi	Wi-Fi
Interoperability	No	No	No

3.4 Telemonitoring Devices Used in Thromboembolic Diseases

Thrombosis is a pathology characterized by excess blood clotting that exists in vessel walls, thus becoming the desirable opposite of homeostasis, where there is coagulation necessary at specific sites of vessels where there is injury. This pathology occurs both in the arterial circulation and in the venous circulation and can trigger different pathologies depending on where it occurs, such as myocardial infarction, pulmonary embolism and ischemic stroke [30].

The possible thromboembolic events are prevented by therapeutic measures such as oral anticoagulants, such as warfarin, and the aim of this therapy is to preserve adjusted anticoagulation levels, preventing events with the lowest possible risk of haemorrhage [31, 32].

The devices described are eCareCompanion, Genesis Telemonitor and Honeywell HomMed. All systems are portable. Honeywell HomMed is the largest platform, thus less easy to transport. Obtaining the INR value is invasive and is performed by puncture to obtain a drop of blood that is placed on a test strip previously placed in an INR monitoring device. In eCareCompanion the value of INR is received via Bluetooth, in the case of Genesis Telemonitor the value is entered manually and in Honeywell HomMed receives the data through a cable connected to the INR monitoring device. Results are sent through Wi-Fi to databases in order to be analysed by specialized health professionals. The patient-to-patient interface is simple and customizable to the patient on all devices [33–35].

Table 4 reviews the technical specifications of devices and telemonitoring systems found for thromboembolic diseases. As in the previous cases, the interoperability between systems and devices is not available.

3.5 Telemonitoring Devices Used in Heart Failure

Heart failure is a disease that is growing in developed countries, despite the diminished incidence of cardiovascular diseases. It is estimated that there are 23

Table 4 Comparison of technical specifications of telemonitoring systems used in Thromboembolic Diseases

	Device 1	Device 2	Device 3
Designation	eCareCompanion	Genesis Telemonitor	Honeywell HomMed
Portability	Yes	Yes	Yes/no
Invasiveness	Yes	Yes	Yes
Interface	Custom and simple	Custom and simple	Custom and simple
Connectivity	Wi-Fi Bluetooth	Wi-Fi Bluetooth 3G/4G	Direct connection to device Wi-Fi
Interoperability	No	No	No

Table 5 Comparison of technical specifications of telemonitoring systems used in Heart Failure

	Device 1	Device 2	Device 3
Designation	VITALS360®	TCare cardio monitor	Smartheart™
Portability	Yes	Yes	Yes
Invasiveness	No	No	No
Interface	Custom and simple	Custom and simple	Custom and simple
Connectivity	Wi-Fi	Bluetooth GSM/HDSPA	BluetoothWi-Fi
Interoperability	No	No	No

million people living with the disease in the world [35, 36]. Due to the progression of the disease, the decompensation is frequent, which leads to hospitalizations also more frequent [37]. In the USA alone, the number of hospitalizations exceeds one million per year, which significantly increases the costs associated with the disease for both the patient and the health system [35]. According to Liu et al. [38, 39], costs directly and indirectly involving the treatment of heart failure in the USA were around $39.2 billion in 2010, with only re-hospitalizations accounting for approximately $31 billion of dollars spent.

The devices described are VITALS360®, TCare Cardio Monitor and Smartheart™. All devices and systems are portable. Obtaining the ECG tracing is non-invasive and is the main test performed with these devices and telemonitoring systems. In VITALS360®, the ECG is performed directly on the device. In the remaining devices, the ECG trace is sent via Bluetooth from external ECG devices. Results are sent through Wi-Fi in the case of TCare Cardio Monitor through GSM/HDSPA. The patient-to-patient interface is simple and customizable to the patient on all devices [12, 40, 41].

Table 5 reviews the technical specifications of the devices and telemonitoring systems found for Heart Failure. Following the path of the telemonitoring devices for the previous pathologies, the interoperability between devices and systems of different brands is inexistent.

4 Proposal for Future Telemonitoring IoT System

The proposed trend-based telemonitoring system is shown in Fig. 1. This is composed of four components (1) wearable monitoring device; (2) smartphone (health application); (3) cloud; (4) call centre, patient and doctor.

The proposal considers a wearable and non-invasive device that is placed in contact with the patient's skin, acquires the indicated biological and physical parameters for the disease in question. The proposed non-invasive wearable monitoring device consists of one or more biological and physical parameter measurement sensors, a microcontroller, a battery and a Bluetooth Low Energy (BLE) integrated circuit. The data is collected by the monitoring device and sent to the smartphone via BLE.

In the smartphone there is a health application that collects and filters firstly the data, according to an algorithm that limits the values. These limits should be adjusted and personalized for each patient, being only sent to the cloud values higher than the reference values. Inter-operation for the remote cloud-based system could be helped by using common health data APIs/wellness data APIs (some of which are already on the market) or health data description taxonomies (currently a focus of research). In the cloud there is another algorithm that decides according to the results received: (1) it communicates some message to the patient. If this condition occurs, an information report is also sent to the specialist doctor who follows the patient. (2) If it is sent to the call centre, the results are outside the limit range and the medical specialists will decide what procedures to take, contact the patient immediately giving instructions of procedures to take, contact the emergency service to move to the patient or even contact the patient's personal doctor to help make a decision.

This ideal IoT telemonitoring system will be able to interoperate with programs developed by different software houses, in order to allow the flow of information of patients' clinical data between healthcare systems at different levels, ensuring the confidentiality and security of data.

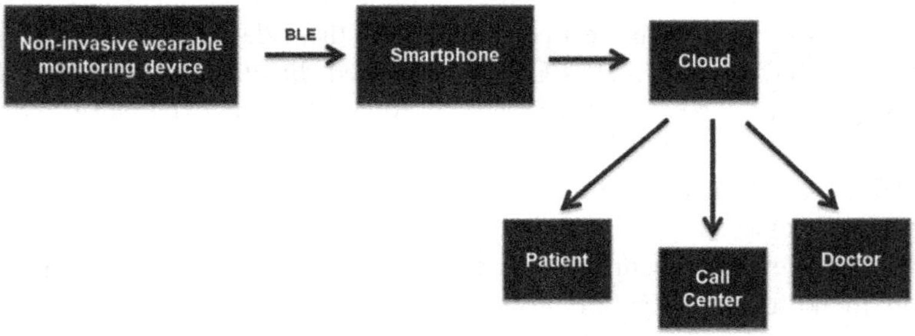

Fig. 1 Scheme of the proposal for future IoT telemonitoring system

5 Conclusions

Telemonitoring for chronic patients can bring great benefits to both the patient and health systems. For the patient the increase of care in the self-management of the disease consequently leads to an improvement in the health condition and quality of life, for the health systems the distribution of resources is achieved in an equitable way reaching the majority of possible chronic population.

The enlargement of this practice applied to chronic pathologies will be a reality in the near future, not forgetting that until this premise becomes real some gaps will have to be overcome as the creation of interoperability programs between health support systems, which is the main failure of the devices and systems telemonitoring existing on the market.

References

1. World Health Organization: Noncommunicable diseases. http://www.who.int/topics/noncommunicable_diseases/en/. Accessed 04 Feb 2017
2. Ho, K.: Supporting heart failure patient transitions from acute to community care with home telemonitoring technology: a protocol for a provincial randomized controlled trial (TEC4Home). JMIR Res. Protoc. **5**(4), e198 (2016)
3. Saner, H., Van Der Velde, E.: eHealth in cardiovascular medicine: a clinical update. Eur. J. Prev. Cardiol. **23**, 5–12 (2016)
4. Paré, G., Moqadem, K., Pineau, G., St-Hilaire, C.: Clinical effects of home telemonitoring in the context of diabetes, asthma, heart failure and hypertension: a systematic review. J. Med. Internet Res. **12**(2), e21 (2010)
5. Esteban, C., Moraza, J., Iriberri, M., Aguirre, U., Goiria, B., Quintana, J.M., Aburto, M., Capelastegui, A.: Outcomes of a telemonitoring-based program (telEPOC) in frequently hospitalized COPD patients. Int. J. COPD. **11**, 2919–2930 (2016)
6. Bashshur, R.L., Shannon, G.W., Smith, B.R., Alverson, D.C., Antoniotti, N., et al.: The empirical foundations of telemedicine interventions for chronic disease management. Telemed. J. E Health. **20**, 769–800 (2014)
7. Gyllensten, I.C., Crundall-Goode, A., Aarts, R.M., Goode, K.M.: Simulated case management of home telemonitoring to assess the impact of different alert algorithms on work-load and clinical decisions. BMC Med. Inform. Decis. Mak. **17**(1), 11 (2017)
8. Craig, M.E., Hattersley, A., Donaghue, K.C.: Definition, epidemiology and classification of diabetes in children and adolescents. Pediatr. Diabetes. **15**, 4–17 (2014)
9. Cariou, B., Eddy, D., Schwarz, P., Gumprecht, J., Smith, U., et al.: The diabetes epidemic and its impact on Europe. In: European Diabetes Leadership Forum, p. 44. OECD, Paris (2012)
10. Wild, S.H., Hanley, J., Lewis, S.C., McKnight, J.A., McCloughan, L.B., et al.: Supported telemonitoring and glycemic control in people with type 2 diabetes: the telescot diabetes pragmatic multicenter randomized controlled trial. PLoS Med. **13**, 1–16 (2016)
11. Edevice: HealthGO Mini. http://www.edevice.com/products/healthgo-mini. Accessed 08 Jun 2017
12. VoCare: Vitals360®. http://vocare.com/vitals360/. Accessed 06 Jun 2017
13. TelehealthSolutions: CareHomePod. https://www.thsl.co.uk/products/carehomepod. Accessed 08 Jun 2017
14. VoCare®. Vitals360® user manual. p. 13 (2013)

15. Pedone, C., Lelli, D.: Systematic review of telemonitoring in copd: an update. Pneumonol. Alergol. Pol. **83**, 476–484 (2015)
16. Vivekanandan, S., Devanand, M.: Remote monitoring for diabetes disorder: pilot study using InDiaTel prototype. Eur. Res. Telemed. **4**, 63–69 (2015)
17. Fitzsimmons, D.A., Thompson, J., Bentley, C.L., Mountain, G.A.: Comparison of patient perceptions of Telehealth-supported and specialist nursing interventions for early stage COPD: a qualitative study. BMC Health Serv. Res. **16**, 420 (2016)
18. Merone, M., Pedone, C., Capasso, G., Incalzi, R.A., Soda, P.: A decision support system for tele-monitoring COPD-related worrisome events. IEEE J. Biomed. Health Informatics. **2194**, 2168–2194 (2017)
19. Mulpuru, S., Mckay, J., Ronksley, P.E., Thavorn, K., Kobewka, D.M., Forster, A.J.: Factors contributing to high-cost hospital care for patients with COPD. Int. J. COPD. **12**, 989–995 (2017)
20. Fonseca, J.A., Costa-Pereira, A., Delgado, L., Silva, L.N., Magalhães, M., Castel-Branco, M.G., Vaz, M.: Pulmonary function electronic monitoring devices: a randomized agreement study. Chest J. **128**, 1258–1265 (2005)
21. Masimo: iSpO2® pulse oximeter. http://masimopersonalhealth.com/products/ispo2-pulse-oximeter/. Accessed 07 Jun 2017
22. Masimo Shop. http://masimopersonalhealth.com/shop/. Accessed 07 Jun 2017
23. Wilson, C., Campbell, S.M., Luker, K.A., Caress, A.L.: Referral and management options for patients with chronic kidney disease: perspectives of patients, generalists and specialists. Health Expect. **18**, 325–334 (2015)
24. Cuevas, J.R., Dominguez, E.L., Velazquez, Y.H.: Telemonitoring system for patients with chronic kidney disease undergoing peritoneal dialysis. IEEE Lat. Am. Trans. **14**, 2000–2006 (2016)
25. Raman, M., Green, D., Middleton, R.J., Kalra, P.A.: Older people with chronic kidney disease: definition, and influence of biomarkers and medications upon cardiovascular and renal outcomes. J. Ren. Care. **42**, 150–161 (2016)
26. Thilly, N., Chanliau, J., Frimat, L., Combe, C., Merville, P., et al.: Cost-effectiveness of home telemonitoring in chronic kidney disease patients at different stages by a pragmatic randomized controlled trial (eNephro): rationale and study design. BMC Nephrol. **18**, 126 (2017)
27. Singh, P., Ricksten, S.E., Bragadottir, G., Redfors, B., Nordquist, L.: Renal oxygenation and haemodynamics in acute kidney injury and chronic kidney disease. Clin. Exp. Pharmacol. Physiol. **40**, 138–147 (2013)
28. Trifirò, G., Fatuzzo, P.M., Ientile, V., Pizzimenti, V., Ferrajolo, C., et al.: Expert opinion of nephrologists about the effectiveness of low-protein diet in different stages of chronic kidney disease (CKD). Int. J. Food Sci. Nutr. **65**, 1027–1032 (2014)
29. eQOL: Our solutions empower patients to manage their care outside of the hospital. https://eqol.ca/index.php (2017). Accessed 11 Jun 2017
30. Jeffs, L., Jain, A.K., Man, R.H., Onabajo, N., Desveaux, L., et al.: Exploring the utility and scalability of a telehomecare intervention for patients with chronic kidney disease undergoing peritoneal dialysis—a study protocol. BMC Nephrol. **18**, 155 (2017)
31. Kenne, E., Nickel, K.F., Long, A.T., Fuchs, T.A., Stavrou, E.X., et al.: Factor XII: a novel target for safe prevention of thrombosis and inflammation. J. Intern. Med. **278**, 571–585 (2015)
32. Araújo, A.C.O., Domingues, R.B., van Bellen, B.: Determinação do INR: Comparação entre método convencional e dispositivo portátil. J. Vasc. Bras. **13**, 88–93 (2014)
33. Philips: eCareCompanion patient app. http://www.usa.philips.com/healthcare/product/HCNOCTN483/ecarecompanion-patient-app-your-patients-gateway-to-care. Accessed 09 Jun 2017
34. Honeywell Life Care: Genesis telemonitor – targeted solution. https://www.honeywelllifecare.com/lifestream-products/legacy-products-and-software/genesis-telemonitor/. Accessed 09 Jun 2017
35. Pyramidhhs. http://pyramidhhs.com/index.php/services/home-health/missouri-telemonitoring-remote-disease-management. Accessed 09 Jun 2017

36. Pyramid HHS. http://pyramidhhs.com/index.php/contact-us. Accessed 09 Jun 2017
37. Tadic, M., Pieske-Kraigher, E., Cuspidi, C., Genger, M., Morris, D.A., et al.: Left ventricular strain and twisting in heart failure with preserved ejection fraction: an updated review. Heart Fail. Rev. **22**, 371–379 (2017)
38. Knox, L., Rahman, R.J., Beedie, C.: Quality of life in patients receiving telemedicine enhanced chronic heart failure disease management: a meta-analysis. J. Telemed. Telecare. **23**(7), 639–649 (2017)
39. Pazos-López, P., Peteiro-Vázquez, J., Carcía-Campos, A., García-Bueno, L., de Torres, J.P.A., Castro-Beiras, A.: The causes, consequences, and treatment of left or right heart failure. Vasc. Health Risk Manag. **7**, 237–254 (2011)
40. TCare Cardio Monitor. http://www.tcare.pt/servicos/tcare-cardio-monitor/. Accessed 04 Jun 2017
41. SHL Telemedicine: SmartHeart. http://www.shl-telemedicine.com/portfolio/smartheart/. Accessed 08 Jun 2017

A Machine Learning Method for Screening Children with Patent Ductus Arteriosus Using Intelligent Phonocardiography

Arash Gharehbaghi, Ankica Babic, and Amir A. Sepehri

1 Introduction

Intelligent phonocardiography as a non-invasive and inexpensive approach has been recently sounded for screening cardiac disease [1, 2]. Recent studies revealed that application of the intelligent phonocardiography is not limited only to screening pediatric heart disease, as it steps toward associating diagnostic value with the approach [3–5]. Importance of this approach is better realized when considering that a large number of the pediatric referrals to the hospital have normal hearts, while shortage of pediatric cardiologists causes long waiting time for the families which brings stress and costs to the healthcare system. On the other hand, there are still a considerable number of pediatric patients in the primary healthcare centers which are negatively misdiagnosed due to the complexities in cardiac auscultation as it is still employed for the screening purpose [6]. Patent ductus arteriosus (PDA) is a congenital disease caused by an abnormal blood flow between the two major arteries exiting the heart. Aortic and pulmonary artery are connected through a vessel, named ductus arteriosus before birth. Although ductus arteriosus plays an important role in fetal blood circulation, it should be naturally ceased within a few hours after the birth when the lung performs a normal respiration. Those children whose ductus arteriosus remains opened long after the birth are considered as suffering

A. Gharehbaghi (✉)
Department of Innovation, Design and Technology, Mälardalen University, Västerås, Sweden
e-mail: arash.ghareh.baghi@mdh.se

A. Babic
Department of Biomedical Engineering, Linköping University, Linköping, Sweden

Department of Information Science and Media Studies, University of Bergen, Bergen, Norway

A. A. Sepehri
CAPIS Biomedical Research and Development Centre, Mons, Belgium

P. R. M. Inácio et al. (eds.), *5th EAI International Conference on IoT Technologies for HealthCare*, EAI/Springer Innovations in Communication and Computing,
https://doi.org/10.1007/978-3-030-30335-8_7

from PDA. A child with untreated PDA can develop complications like pulmonary hypertension which may require heart or lung transplant in the long term. It is therefore of critical importance to screen children with PDA soon before developing serious complications when the disease progress can be controlled by an appropriate management. One of the manifestations of PDA is a continuous heart murmur heard in both the systole and the diastole. Auscultation of the murmur initiated by a PDA is a complicated task, especially for the unexperienced practitioners and nurses of primary healthcare centers. Studies on the intelligent phonocardiography toward murmur classification in children have been profoundly reported over decades [7–10]. However, this is not true for developing a sophisticated processing method for screening children with PDA from the heart sound signal. This paper presents a novel method for processing heart sound signals to detect PDA murmur. The method adjusts our internationally patented method (PCT/EP2009/051410), which we called the Arash-Band, in a way to include temporal characteristics of the signal. Results showed an acceptable performance for the classification comparing to the one for a practitioner which had been reported to be below 70%. The method exhibits low complexities in testing, offering the possibility to be used either as a decision support in the primary healthcare centers or as a distributed screening system on the web technology [11].

2 Materials and Methods

2.1 The Data Preparation

Heart sound signal and electrocardiogram (ECG) were recorded from 50 children, who referred to Children Medical Centre of Tehran University, Iran, using an electronic stethoscope of Meditron Analyzer in conjunction with a DELL laptop equipped with 16-bit sound card. The sampling rate was 44,100 Hz to have good recording/play back signal. Each recording had 10 s duration. All the referrals gave the informed consent for participating in the study. The study was conducted according to the Good Clinical Practice, and complied with World Medical Association and Declaration of Helsinki, and approved by the institutional committee of ethics. All the referrals were examined by a pediatric cardiologist who used echocardiography as the gold standard in companion with the ECG, chest X-ray, and other complementary tests. The patient population is listed in Table 1.

2.2 The Processing Method

The heart sound signals were downsampled using an anti-aliasing filter and segmented through which the first and the second heart sounds were carefully annotated

Table 1 The patient characteristics of the participating population

Total number of patients	50
Number of healthy individuals with no murmur	15
Number of healthy individuals with innocent murmur	15
Age range of the healthy individuals	4–15 years
Number of patients with patent ductus arteriosus	20
Age range of the patients with patent ductus arteriosus	0–5 years

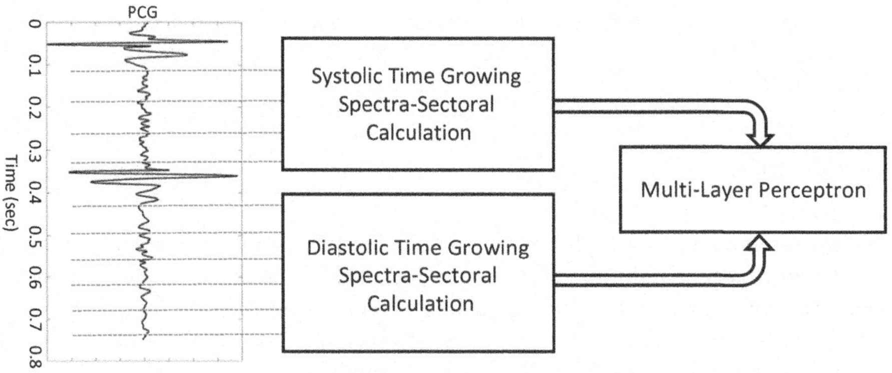

Fig. 1 An illustration of the innovative processing method. Details of the calculations can be found in [12]

according to the concurrence with the ECG peaks. The processing method is based on our original method, named Short Time Arash-Band, which relies on spectral calculation over two sets of the short sectors of the signal, one set for processing the systolic and the other set for the diastolic parts, independently. Then, the spectra-sectoral contents of the signal are calculated for the purpose of feature selection. Details of the spectra-sectoral calculations are found in [12]. Figure 1 illustrates the sectoral processing. A backward growing with three sectors and a forward growing with five sectors are empirically selected to analyze the systolic and diastolic parts of the signal, respectively. The spectral contents of the sectors are calculated using the priodogram. For each sector, a discriminative frequency band is found based on the Arash-Band method [12]. The calculated spectra-sectoral energies are employed by a multilayer perceptron neural network for the classification.

2.3 The Evaluation

Performance of the method is evaluated by using leave-one-out method. In this method, one single data is used for testing the method and the rest for training.

This procedure is repeated 50 times with each single recording used only once for testing. Then, the accuracy of the method is calculated as:

$$P_{ac} = 100\frac{N_{TP} + N_{TN}}{N_{TP} + N_{TN} + N_{FP} + N_{FN}} \quad (1)$$

where N_{TN} and N_{TP} are the number of the correctly classified individuals from the healthy and the PDA groups, respectively. The N_{FP} and N_{FN} are the number of the incorrectly classified individuals from the PDA and the healthy groups, respectively. The leave-one-out method is suitable when the data size is small, as is the case for this study.

3 Results

Figure 2 demonstrates samples of the healthy and PDA group. The healthy subject shows an innocent murmur, whereas for the PDA the murmur is of continuous one. The murmur intensity of the healthy subject is heard even higher than the PDA patient. This makes the differentiation problematic using both the conventional auscultation and the artificial intelligent-based methods.

Figure 3 demonstrates result of the leave-one-out method, applied to the 50 signals of our database.

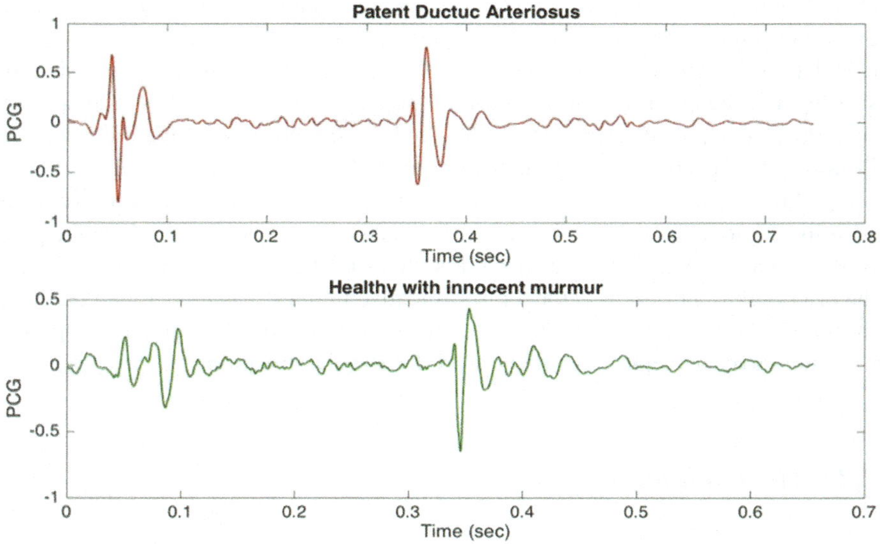

Fig. 2 A sample of the healthy subject (with innocent murmur) against another one with PDA, from our database

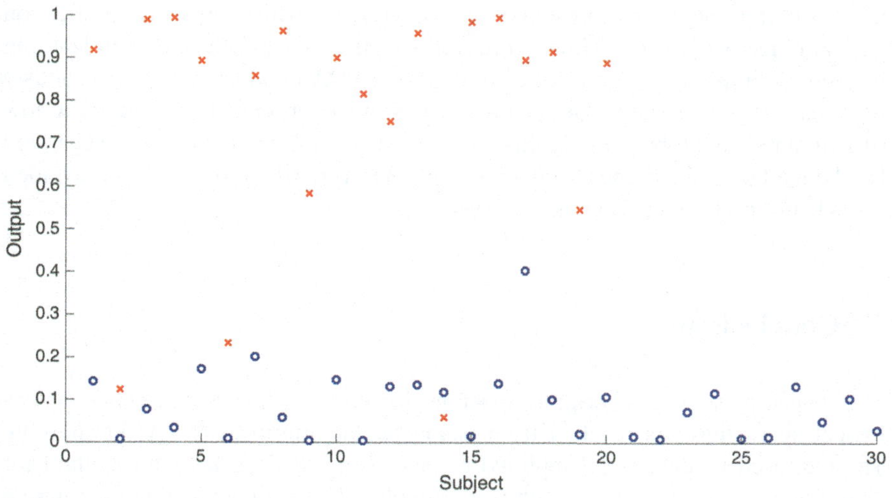

Fig. 3 Output of the method for the healthy children (blue **O**) and the children with patent ductus arteriosus (red **X**)

As can be seen, the two groups are acceptably segregated using the proposed method. However, there are three children with PDA which are misdiagnosed by the method, offering a sensitivity of 85%. All the three false negative patients are subjects of silent PDA, which can be considered as healthy individuals. Referring to the database, all the three patients have small PDA. On the other hand, there are four cases of healthy children which are classified as abnormal, because of the high intensity innocent murmur. These individuals mostly undergo echocardiography. The accuracy of the method is estimated to be 86% with a specificity of 87%.

4 Discussion

This paper suggested the intelligent phonocardiography as an automated approach for improving screening accuracy of the children with congenital heart disease in primary healthcare centers. The approach is easy-to-use, inexpensive, non-invasive, and quick that allows the practitioners and nurses to candidate proper patients to undergo echocardiography. The processing method proposed in this paper is based on the advanced deep learning method [12], but with an empirical modification toward more simplification for a quick learning. Although the advanced deep learning method shows minimal structural risk compared to a hybrid method [13], complexity of the presented method in this paper also is minimal in the both training and testing phase. The suggested method takes both the temporal and spectral contents of the heart sound into consideration such that an optimal classification is obtained. Application of artificial neural networks had been reported in a large number of the studies on heart sound signal analysis, in which murmur classification was an objective [14–19]. However, development of a sophisticated deep learning method, with minimal complexities in detecting PDA children was not previously reported. One of the important characteristics of the presented method is the low structural risk and robustness against the test data [12]. Nevertheless, it is necessary for the method to be trained with a broader dataset by which overfitting is avoided and a better performance can be observed.

5 Conclusions

This paper presented an original machine learning method for detecting pathological heart murmurs resulted from patent ductus arteriosus (PDA) in children. The purposed method is a simplified extension of our deep learning method for classifying cyclic time series, with a considerably less complexities in the training phase. Results of the leave-one-out validation method exhibited an acceptable performance, outperforming a typical pediatrician who employs conventional auscultation. The method can be easily integrated with a portable computer to be used as an efficient decision support system in primary healthcare centers.

Acknowledgments This study was supported by the CAPIS Inc., Mons, Belgium, and also by the KKS financed research profile in embedded sensor systems for health at Mälardalen University, Västerås, Sweden.

Conflict of Interest The authors declare that they have no conflict of interest.

References

1. Gharehbaghi, A., Ekman, I., Ask, P., Nylander, E., Janerot-Sjöberg, B.: Assessment of aortic valve stenosis using intelligent phonocardiography. Int. J. Cardiol. **198**, 58–60 (2015)
2. Gharehbaghi, A., Dutoit, T., Sepehri, A.A., Kocharian, A., Lindén, M.: A novel method for screening children with isolated bicuspid aortic valve. Cardiovasc. Eng. Technol. **6**(4), 546–556 (2015)
3. Gharehbaghi, A., Ask, P., Nylander, E., Janerot-Sjöberg, B., Ekman, I., Lindén, M., Babic, A.: A hybrid model for diagnosing sever aortic stenosis in asymptomatic patients using phonocardiogram. In: World Congress on Medical Physics and Biomedical Engineering, Toronto, Canada, pp. 1006–1009. Springer, Cham (2015)
4. Gharehbaghi, A., Sepehri, A.A., Kocharian, A., Lindén, M.: An intelligent method for discrimination between aortic and pulmonary stenosis using phonocardiogram. In: World Congress on Medical Physics and Biomedical Engineering, Toronto, Canada, pp. 1010–1013. Springer, Cham (2015)
5. Gharehbaghi, A., Sepehri, A.A., Lindén, M., Babic, A.: Intelligent phonocardiography for screening ventricular septal defect using time growing neural network. In: Mantas, J., Hasman, G., Gallos, G. (eds.) Informatics Empowers Healthcare Transformation, pp. 108–111. IOS Press, Amsterdam (2017)

6. Watrous, R.L., Thompson, W.R., Ackerma, S.J.: The impact of computer-assisted auscultation on physician referrals of asymptomatic patients with heart murmurs. Clin. Cardiol. **31**(2), 79–83 (2008)
7. Akay, Y.M., Akay, M., Welkowitz, W., Semmlow, J.L., Kostis, J.B.: Noninvasive acoustical detection of coronary artery disease: a comparative study of signal processing methods. IEEE Trans. Biomed. Eng. **40**(6), 571–578 (1993)
8. Gharehbaghi, A., Sepehri, A.A., Lindén, M., Babic, A.: A hybrid machine learning method for detecting cardiac ejection murmurs. In: EMBEC & NBC 2017, pp. 787–790. Springer, Singapore (2017)
9. Gharehbaghi, A., Lindén, M., Babic, A.: A decision support system for cardiac disease diagnosis based on machine learning methods. In: Informatics for Health: Connected Citizen-Led Wellness and Population Health, pp. 235–238. IOS Press, Amsterdam (2017)
10. Welkowitz, W., Akay, M., Wang, J.Z., Semmlow, J., Kotis, J.: A model for distributed coronary artery flow with phonocardiography verification. Card. Electrophys. Circ. Transp. **121**, 261–272 (1991)
11. Gharehbaghi, A., Lindén, M.: An internet-based tool for pediatric cardiac disease diagnosis using intelligent phonocardiography. In: Internet of Things. IoT Infrastructures: Second International Summit, IoT 360°, Rome, Italy, pp. 443–447. Springer, Cham (2015)
12. Gharehbaghi, A., Lindén, M.: A deep machine learning method for classifying cyclic time series of biological signals using time-growing neural network. IEEE Trans. Neural Netw. Learn. Syst. **29**(9), 4102–4115 (2018)
13. Gharehbaghi, A., Babic, A.: Structural risk evaluation of a deep neural network and a Markov Model in extracting medical information from phonocardiography. Stud. Health Technol. Inform. **251**, 157–160 (2018)
14. DeGroff, C.G., et al.: Artificial neural network-based method of screening heart murmurs in children. Circulation. **103**, 2711–2716 (2001)
15. Sinha, R.K., et al.: Backpropagation artificial neural network classifier to detect changes in heart sound due to mitral valve regurgitation. J. Med. Syst. **31**, 205–209 (2007)
16. Ari, S., et al.: In search of an optimization technique for artificial neural network to classify abnormal heart sounds. Appl. Soft Comput. **9**, 330–340 (2009)
17. Dokure, Z., et al.: Heart sound classification using wavelet transform and incremental self-organizing map. Digit. Signal Process. **18**, 951–959 (2008)
18. Gharehbaghi, A., Babic, A., Sepehri, A.A.: Extraction of diagnostic information from phonocardiographic signal using time-growing neural network. In: World Congress on Medical Physics and Biomedical Engineering, pp. 849–853. Springer, Singapore (2019)
19. Sepehri, A.A., Kocharian, A., Janani, A., Gharehbaghi, A.: An intelligent phonocardiography for automated screening of pediatric heart diseases. J. Med. Syst. **40**, 16 (2016)

Internet-of-Things Based Respiratory Rate Monitoring for Early Detection of Cardiovascular and Pulmonary Diseases

Amaia Soubelet, Rahul Krishnan Pathinarupothi, Ekanath Srihari Rangan, Kripesh, P. Durga, and K. A. Unnikrishna Menon

1 Introduction

Cardiovascular and pulmonary diseases are the leading causes of death in many developed and developing parts of the world, with a total of 21% and 19% of annual deaths attributed to these, respectively, in the age group of 25–69 years [1]. It is widely acknowledged that the problem of increasing risk factors for cardiovascular and pulmonary diseases is the lack of surveillance system for timely diagnosis [2]. These challenges are acutely amplified in rural and remote regions, where there is a startling lack of accessibility to healthcare facilities due to which villagers do not generally go for regular health checkups. Apart from the lack of accessibility, many villagers cannot afford to visit far away specialty hospitals to see a physician, unless critically ill.

One of the promising technological solutions that can potentially bring about a marked change in this situation is the use of Internet-of-Things (IoT) based remote health monitoring (RHM). Our research group at Amrita University in collaboration

This project was supported in part through funding from the Department of Science and Technology, Govt. of India, grant no. IDP/MED/10/2015. First and second authors have contributed equally to this work.

A. Soubelet (✉)
Ecole Polytechnique Fédérale de Lausanne, Lausanne, Switzerland

R. K. Pathinarupothi · Kripesh · P. Durga · K. A. U. Menon
Amrita Center for Wireless Networks and Applications (AmritaWNA), Amrita School of Engineering, Amritapuri, Amrita Vishwa Vidyapeetham, Vallikavu, Kerala, India
e-mail: rahulkrishnan@am.amrita.edu

E. S. Rangan
Amrita School of Medicine, Kochi, Amrita Vishwa Vidyapeetham, Kochi, Kerala, India

P. R. M. Inácio et al. (eds.), *5th EAI International Conference on IoT Technologies for HealthCare*, EAI/Springer Innovations in Communication and Computing,
https://doi.org/10.1007/978-3-030-30335-8_8

with our large University hospital, Amrita Institute of Medical Sciences (AIMS), India, has developed an IoT based RHM system in which patients use a body worn IoT device that includes ECG and photoplethysmograph (PPG) sensors that continuously monitor their electrocardiograph (ECG), pulse rate (PR), respiratory rate (RR), blood pressure (BP), and blood oxygen (SpO2) [3]. A patient wears this device all day long on his/her wrist and the vital parameters are sent to physicians in specialty hospitals over the cloud or directly to their smartphones as and when required. The parameters sent from this device are used to monitor and detect, early on, many cardiovascular, pulmonary, and neurological disorders such as cardiac arrest, cardiac arrhythmias, sleep apnea, hypertension and stroke, pneumonia, chronic obstructive pulmonary disease, etc.

Along with the other vital parameters, respiratory rate (RR) is one of the most clinically relevant parameters that can diagnose and monitor the severity of many pulmonary, metabolic, neurological, and cardiovascular diseases. Moreover, the possibility of monitoring RR along with other vitals using small wearables increases the prospects of extending critical care to peripheral centers and subcritical care to homes. Some of the diseases that warrant such monitoring include metabolic acidosis (a complication of diabetes), acute respiratory distress syndrome, pneumothorax, acute asthma, pneumonia, chronic obstructive pulmonary disease (COPD), etc. These conditions can result in a type of respiratory failure wherein there is hypoxia (low PaO2) and Tachypnea. Some of the chronic lung diseases, including sleep apnea, could result in hypertrophy and failure of the right ventricle of the heart. Another very pragmatic application is the use of RR for identification and classification of pneumonia in children, according to the WHO clinical classification criteria: (a) 2–12 months: RR > =50/min, (b) 1–5 years: RR > =40/min, and (c) 6 years and above: RR > =20/min. The role of RR estimates in early detection of many critical diseases as well as the ease with which wearable sensors can be used to obtain PPG signals (which are modulated by respiratory signals), makes it even more important to have robust algorithms for automated RR estimation from PPG signals. Hence, in this paper, we particularly focus on such algorithms that automatically estimate RR from PPG signals.

Our paper contributes the following:

- A review of existing reported work on RR measurement from PPG signals and their performances.
- A real-world validation of a PPG based IoT sensor on 25 subjects, for computation of RR.
- A comparison of 15 different processing algorithms for RR derivation from PPG signals.

The rest of this paper is organized as follows: In Sect. 2, we begin with a review of related work. In Sect. 3, we describe our system architecture. We detail the experimentation design, the sensor device, algorithms used, and data collection procedure in Sect. 4. We present our validation study results in Sect. 5, and finally we conclude this paper in Sect. 6.

2 Related Work

Addison et al. [4] estimated the respiratory rate using an algorithm based on continuous wavelet transform technology within an infrastructure incorporating weighted averaging and logical decision-making processes. The correlation coefficient between this method and an end-tidal CO2 reference rate is reported as 0.93. Garde et al. [5] employed an algorithm based on the correntropy spectral density (CSD) to estimate the respiratory rate. They tested the algorithm against the CapnoBase benchmark dataset [6]. It gave them an unnormalized root mean square error of 0.95 breaths/min and a median error of 4.2 breaths/min when using 60 s windows and 1.9 breaths/min when using 120 s windows. The median error significantly decreased ($p < 0.05$) with longer time windows when CSD (from 1.77 to 0.95 breaths/min) approach was employed.

Madhav et al. [7] created an algorithm called modified multiscale principal component analysis to estimate the respiratory rate from PPG signals. The number of data set used in this paper is 15 healthy subjects and the reported accuracy was 98%. Lin et al. [8] estimated the respiratory rate from the PPG signal using a wavelet-based algorithm (the complex Morlet wavelet). They conducted an experiment with five healthy subjects. The correlation coefficient between the respiratory rate derived from PPG signal and respiratory signal is 0.9678. Nilsson et al. [9] used a third order Butterworth Band-pass filter with a pass-band from 0.1 to 0.3 Hz. The obtained average error is <0.5 breaths/min when compared to the reference rate, with a correlation of 0.93. These works present a representative set of the broad research literature that is available in the area [10, 11]. We summarize and compare these techniques in Table 1.

Table 1 Comparative analysis of different methods to estimate respiratory rate from PPG

Work	Methods	Sample characteristics	Results
Addison et al. [4]	Continuous wavelet transform	139 healthy adults (58 M, 81 F)	Correlation = 0.93
Garde et al. [5]	Correntropy spectral density	59 children (median age: 8.7) and 35 adults (median age: 52.4)	Error = 1.77–0.95 breaths/min
Madhav et al. [7]	Modified multiscale principal component analysis	15 healthy subjects, age group of 32.5 ± 3.8 (nine male and six female)	Accuracy = 98%
Lin et al. [8]	Wavelet	5 healthy subjects (male, aged 24 ± 1 years)	Error = 0.2534 breaths/min
Nilsson et al. [9]	Third order Butterworth band-pass filter	16 healthy subjects	Error = <0.5 breaths/min Correlation = 0.93

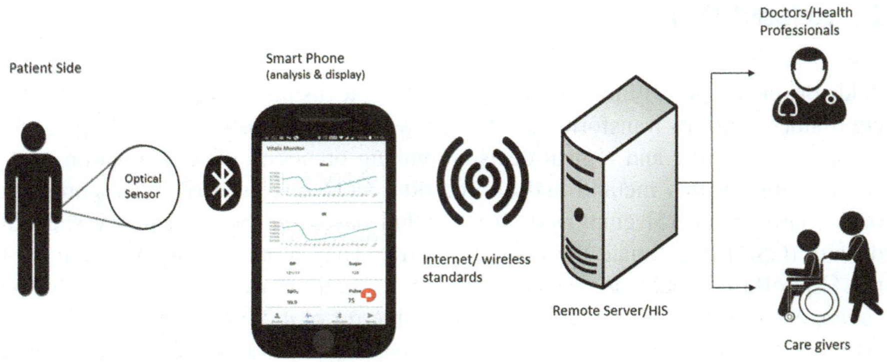

Fig. 1 System architecture showing the transmission of PPG signal from the patient's body to the doctors via mobile app interfaced with the Hospital Information System (HIS) cloud server

3 System Architecture

Our system architecture (see Fig. 1) incorporates different sections, namely sensors and visualization application on the patient side, wireless transmission from the smartphones to the remote server, and the applications running on this remote server. On the patient side, an optical sensor collects PPG signals from a patient's finger-tip, which is used as the primary signal for respiratory rate estimation. The PPG signals are transmitted from the sensor to the patient's smartphone using the Bluetooth Low Energy (BLE) module equipped in the sensor platform. An Android application receives the PPG data, and derives three different vital parameters: pulse rate (PR), blood oxygen (SpO2), and respiratory rate (RR). The values of these parameters are displayed on the smartphone for user assessment, and it is also send to remote hospital information system (HIS) over the internet. Later, a medical expert or caregiver can make use of this information for analysis of a patient, who can then be given advice or prescription remotely. In this paper, we particularly focus on RR estimation from the PPG signals.

4 Experimental Evaluation

4.1 Sensor Device

We used a commercially available off-the-shelf IoT PPG sensor device from Maxim [12] to collect the PPG signals from volunteers. This sensor platform, called Maxim MAXREFDES100#, has multiple health and environment monitoring sensors, including one pulse oximeter that we use in our application. This device uses photoplethysmogram (PPG) based sensor to obtain reflected PPG signal. By using a pulse oximeter which illuminates the skin, it can measure the light reflected by

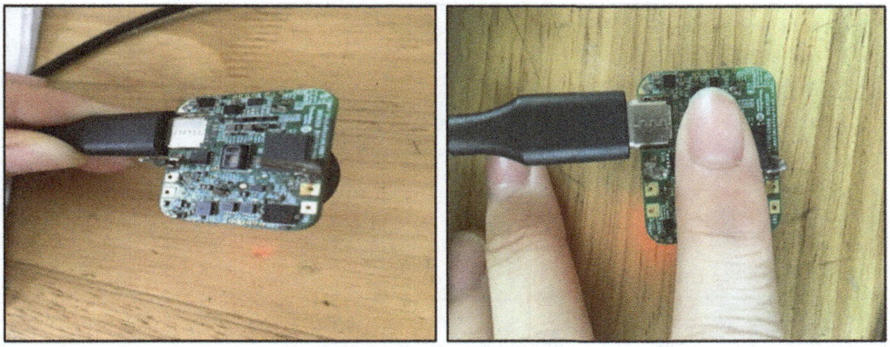

Fig. 2 The Maxim PPG sensor platform that was used for experimentation and data collection

the blood, and generate PPG waveforms in infrared and red regions of the spectrum. Using these signals, we derive RR.

We also used Maxim's Health Sensor Platform for visualization and storage of the PPG signal in a PC. This platform also allows the PPG sensor signal to be stored in a csv file format, which enabled us to use the data for further processing. Figure 2 shows the Maxim PPG sensor device as well how the volunteers used it during our experimentation. Figure 3 shows the screenshot of the user interface that visualizes the PPG signal as well as provides options to tweak the sensor device parameters.

4.2 Algorithms for Computing RR

Once the PPG signals are collected, it needs to be processed in three steps: (a) extraction of the respiratory signal from the PPG signal, (b) calculation of RR from the extracted respiratory signal, and (c) refining RR estimates. These three steps to compute respiratory rates are described below:

Extraction of Respiratory Signal The respiratory activity causes the PPG signal to be modulated in three fundamental ways: through baseline wandering, amplitude modulation, and/or frequency modulation. For the first step, i.e., extraction of the respiratory signal from the PPG signal, we employed two broad approaches: (a) feature based (see Table 2) and (b) filter based (see Table 3) techniques. These techniques are described by Charlton et al. [13]. They had tested these techniques on 57 healthy young subjects aged between 18 and 40 years and elderly subjects aged over 70 years. The correlation coefficient of the respiratory rate measured using gold-standard device and the one calculated using PPG was found to be 0.86 in their experiments. We used a publicly available toolkit [20] that provides a Matlab program to compare these different techniques, and adapted it to make it suitable for our data.

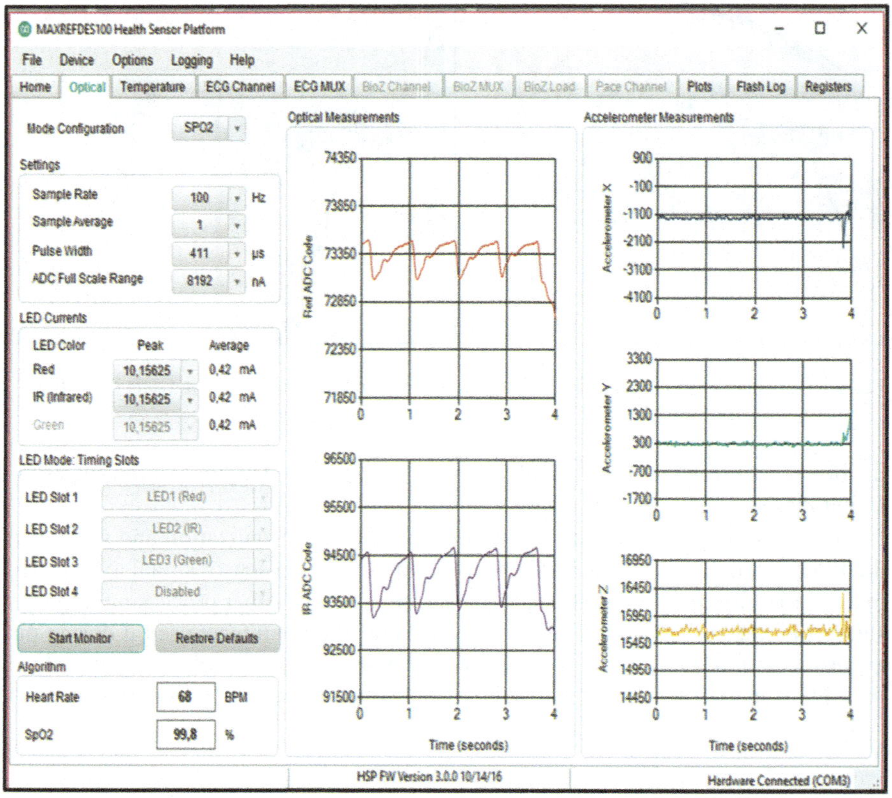

Fig. 3 Screenshot of the front-end software used for visualization of the PPG signals

Table 2 The feature based techniques used for extraction of respiratory signal from PPG signal (adapted from Charlton et al. [13])

Feature based processing	
XB1 (BW)	Mean amplitude of troughs and proceeding peaks (Charlton et al. [13])
XB2 (AM)	Difference between the amplitudes of troughs and proceeding peaks (Karlen et al. [14])
XB3 (FM)	Time interval between consecutive peaks (Karlen et al. [14])
XB4 (BW)	Mean signal value between consecutive troughs (Ruangsuwana et al. [15])
XB5 (BW, AM)	Peak amplitude (Karlen et al. [14])
XB6 (BW, AM)	Trough amplitude (Ruangsuwana et al. [15])
XB9 (BW)	Kernel principal component analysis using a radial basis function, with the variance of the Gaussian kernel determined by maximizing the difference between the first eigenvalue and sum of the remainder (Widjaja et al. [16])
XB10 (FM)	PPG pulse width estimated using a wave boundary detection algorithm (Lázaro et al. [17])

Table 3 The filter based techniques used for extraction of respiratory signal from PPG signal (adapted from Charlton et al. [13])

Filter based processing	
XA1 (BW)	Band-pass filter between plausible respiratory frequencies (Lindberg et al. [18])
XA2 (AM)	The maximum amplitude of the continuous wavelet transform (CWT) within plausible cardiac frequencies (30–220 beats/min) (Addison [19])
XA3 (FM)	The frequency corresponding to the maximum amplitude of the CWT within plausible cardiac frequencies (Addison [19])

Estimation of Respiratory Rate After the respiratory signal is extracted, we employed either one of the two techniques for computation of the respiratory rates: (a) Count Orig—estimates the RR using an implementation of Count Orig [21], and (b) FTS—calculates the frequency spectrum of a signal using FFT (Fast Fourier Transform).

Fusion Techniques for Better Respiratory Rate Estimates Two data fusion techniques, namely Smart Fusion [14] and temporal fusion, were used to further improve the quality of the extracted RR signals.

5 Result and Analysis

We conducted the validation of the wearable IoT device and the above described algorithms with the help of 25 volunteers (12 female and 13 male) in the age group of 23–30 years. First, the volunteers had to sit on a chair and rest for 2 min. Then they have to place their right index finger on the PPG sensor device for 2 min. We did not use any external device to measure the reference respiratory rate, and hence, each subject was asked to mentally count the number of breathing cycles that they took during these 2 min. This count was then entered into the program as the reference rate.

Once all the data was collected, we used a Matlab program [20] to analyze the performance of different algorithms in deriving RR from the PPG signals. The performance of algorithms was compared against the reference RR, and we report the mean absolute error (MAE) as the evaluation parameter.

5.1 Modulation

The algorithms based on frequency modulation (FM) suited best for 8 subjects (MAE = 0.29 breaths/min) as against for six based on amplitude modulation (AM) (MAE = 0.37 breaths/min), five on baseline wandering (BW) (MAE = 0.70 breaths/min), and six on combination of the modulations (MAE = 0.9 breaths/min).

5.2 Feature Based Vs. Filter Based

In general, the least MAE was observed for algorithms which used feature based techniques for respiratory signal extraction. Of the 25 volunteers, 22 gave the best results for feature based techniques, whereas three had the best results using filter based techniques. However, we observed that for different subjects, different feature based algorithms gave the best performance. In 22 subjects in whom the feature based techniques performed the best, the average MAE was 0.54 breaths/min. While for three subjects in whom the filter based technique performed the best, the MAE was 1.3 breaths/min.

5.3 Respiratory Rate Estimation

In the second step, i.e., estimation of the respiratory rate, Count Orig [21] gave best performance on 14 volunteers (with average MAE = 0.58 breaths/min), whereas FFT based technique showed least errors in the rest of 11 subjects (with average MAE = 0.69 breath/min).

In the third step, i.e., fusion of different respiratory signals for further refinement of the results, we observed that out of the 25 subjects, 18 showed improved results using Smart Fusion ($N = 5$) and temporal fusion ($N = 13$).

5.4 Discussion

From these results, we observe that feature based techniques are comparatively better in the extraction of RR signals from the PPG signals, and Count Orig algorithm performs marginally better RR estimation in the subsequent step. These observations are largely corroborated in other studies as well, and our real-world validation using an IoT device provides stronger support to the already existing evidence in this domain.

Since the subjects had to count themselves the number of breath they took during the 2 min of experimentation, it is highly probable that some of the subjects might have made errors in counting. They may also have moved their fingers during the experiment, which might have caused some noise in the PPG signal. The first problem could be solved by using gold-standard devices for measuring RR. The second problem could be solved using a finger-clip that keeps the sensor tightly fixed to the index finger, giving little chance for any movement noise to creep into the PPG signal.

6 Conclusion and Future Work

In this work, we set out to use a single PPG sensor device to derive respiratory rate of patients. We report that the best methods for extraction of respiratory signal from PPG signal are based on feature based techniques, and Count Orig algorithm performed best in respiratory rate estimation. We believe that this is one of the first steps of estimating respiratory rate precisely, using PPG signals. With this single sensor and corresponding software algorithms, people in remote villages will be able to monitor their respiration rate which could be sent to their doctors remotely. This device and the algorithms have far reaching impact in detecting and potentially preventing many NCDs like pneumonia, sleep apnea, or chronic respiratory diseases. This could also drastically improve the early diagnosis and health monitoring of children in remote areas, thereby reducing the child morbidity and mortality rates.

References

1. Web link: https://www.cdc.gov/globalhealth/countries/india/default.htm
2. Nag, T., Ghosh, A.: Cardiovascular disease risk factors in Asian Indian population: a systematic review. J. Cardiovasc. Dis. Res. **4**(4), 222–228 (2013)
3. Pathinarupothi, R.K., Durga, P., Rangan, E.S.: IoT based smart edge for global health: remote monitoring with severity detection and alerts transmission. IEEE Internet Things J. **6**(2), 2449–2462 (2018)
4. Addison, P.S., Watson, J.N., Mestek, M.L., Mecca, R.S.: Developing an algorithm for pulse oximetry derived respiratory rate (RRoxi): a healthy volunteer study. J. Clin. Monit. Comput. **26**(1), 45–51 (2012)
5. Garde, A., Karlen, W., Ansermino, J.M., Dumont, G.A.: Estimating respiratory and heart rates from the correntropy spectral density of the photoplethysmogram. PLoS One. **9**(1), e86427 (2014)
6. Web link: http://www.capnobase.org/database/pulse-oximeter-ieee-tbme-benchmark/
7. Madhav, K.V., Ram, M.R., Krishna, E.H., Komalla, N.R., Reddy, K.A.: Robust extraction of respiratory activity f—-rom PPG signals using modified MSPCA. IEEE Trans. Instrum. Meas. **62**(5), 1094–1106 (2013)
8. Lin, Y.D., Chien, Y.H., Chen, Y.S.: Wavelet-based embedded algorithm for respiratory rate estimation from PPG signal. Biomed. Signal Process. Control. **36**, 138–145 (2017)
9. Nilsson, L., Goscinski, T., Johansson, A., Lindberg, L.G., Kalman, S.: Age and gender do not influence the ability to detect respiration by photoplethysmography. J. Clin. Monit. Comput. **20**(6), 431–436 (2006)
10. Garbhapu, V.V., Gopalan, S.: IoT based low cost single sensor node remote health monitoring system. Procedia Comput. Sci. **113**, 408–415 (2017)
11. Rajevenceltha, J., Kumar, C.S., Kumar, A.A.: Improving the performance of multi-parameter patient monitors using feature mapping and decision fusion. In: Region 10 Conference (TENCON), 2016 IEEE, pp. 1515–1518. IEEE (2016)
12. Web link: https://www.maximintegrated.com/en/design/reference-design-center/system-board/6312.html

13. Charlton, P.H., Bonnici, T., Tarassenko, L., Alastruey, J., Clifton, D.A., Beale, R., Watkinson, P.J.: Extraction of respiratory signals from the electrocardiogram and photoplethysmogram: technical and physiological determinants. Physiol. Meas. **38**(5), 669 (2017)
14. Karlen, W., Raman, S., Ansermino, J.M., Dumont, G.A.: Multiparameter respiratory rate estimation from the photoplethysmogram. IEEE Trans. Biomed. Eng. **60**(7), 1946–1953 (2013)
15. Ruangsuwana, R., Velikic, G., Bocko, M.: Methods to extract respiration information from ECG signals. In: Acoustics Speech and Signal Processing (ICASSP), 2010 IEEE International Conference on, pp. 570–573. IEEE (2010)
16. Widjaja, D., Varon, C., Dorado, A., Suykens, J.A., Van Huffel, S.: Application of kernel principal component analysis for single-lead-ECG-derived respiration. IEEE Trans. Biomed. Eng. **59**(4), 1169–1176 (2012)
17. Lázaro Plaza, J., Bailón Luesma, R., Laguna Lasaosa, P., Gil Herrando, E.: Non-invasive techniques for respiratory information extraction based on pulse photoplethysmogram and electrocardiogram. Doctoral dissertation, Universidad de Zaragoza, Prensas de la Universidad (2015)
18. Lindberg, L.G., Ugnell, H., Öberg, P.Å.: Monitoring of respiratory and heart rates using a fibre-optic sensor. Med. Biol. Eng. Comput. **30**(5), 533–537 (1992)
19. Addison, P.S., Watson, J.N.: Secondary transform decoupling of shifted nonstationary signal modulation components: application to photoplethysmography. Int. J. Wavelets Multiresolution Inf. Process. **2**(01), 43–57 (2004)
20. Link to source code: http://peterhcharlton.github.io/RRest/
21. Schäfer, A., Kratky, K.W.: Estimation of breathing rate from respiratory sinus arrhythmia: comparison of various methods. Ann. Biomed. Eng. **36**(3), 476 (2008)

An Exergame Integrated with IoT to Support Remote Rehabilitation

Kyle Mulholland and Sari Merilampi

1 Introduction

As the proportion of the world's population in older ages continues to increase, the need for improved strategies in provision of healthcare arises. In Finland, the ageing population percentage is continually increasing. Predictions indicate that by 2060 almost one-third of the population will be 65 years and older [1]. This trend represents a global phenomenon with profound implications worldwide [2].

As a significant percentage of the population ages, the respective burden of care and associated demand on the healthcare system increases. As this occurs, existing healthcare facilities, organisations and resources will become increasingly stretched [3]. Leveraging emerging technologies such as IoT within the field of healthcare offers a potential mechanism to combat this growing problem.

IoT capabilities have evolved in recent years, fueled by the prevalence of devices enabled by open wireless technology. It is estimated that by 2020, the number of interconnected devices will reach 24 billion [4]. Ubiquitous and pervasive technologies such as Bluetooth, Wi-Fi, radio frequency identification (RFID) and other wireless communication technologies have facilitated this growing development [5].

With the emergence of IoT, opportunities arise within the healthcare and rehabilitation sector. Healthcare is considered one of the most important application areas of IoT, offering the potential for enhanced health management systems through efficient collection and analysis of patient data for a range of physiological parameters [6]. IoT-based healthcare technologies may also facilitate automation of medical intervention (for example, automating delivery of insulin for individuals with diabetes) and scheduling of limited resources [6, 7]. Accordingly, there are

K. Mulholland (✉) · S. Merilampi
Satakunta University of Applied Sciences, Pori, Finland
e-mail: kyle.2.mulholland@samk.fi

P. R. M. Inácio et al. (eds.), *5th EAI International Conference on IoT Technologies for HealthCare*, EAI/Springer Innovations in Communication and Computing,
https://doi.org/10.1007/978-3-030-30335-8_9

numerous potential benefits associated with the incorporation of IoT technologies into healthcare, with positive outcomes already demonstrated in real-time monitoring, patient information administration, medical emergency management and blood information management [7].

From a review of the latest IoT-based healthcare applications, the most immediate use for IoT technology in healthcare appears to be aimed at ensuring adherence [7]. This represents a topic of great concern, particularly when considering intervention and rehabilitation. Rehabilitation protocols and associated HEP are important instruments in the delivery of successful healthcare interventions, especially within the physiotherapeutic setting. Research indicates that adherence to HEP can be effective in reducing mortality, falls and injuries [8]. Unfortunately, it has also been demonstrated that as little as 35% of patients complete prescribed home exercise with full adherence [9].

One potential method for promoting adherence to HEP involves the use of gamification. Game orientated exercise, or exergames, has been reported as a fun and motivating tool that may increase adherence to HEP [8]. Although more extensive research is required on this topic, studies indicate positive retention and adherence rates concerning effectiveness and feasibility of exergaming systems in the remote or home rehabilitation setting [8].

Emerging tools and technologies such as exergames and IoT possess the ability to serve as complementary tools in the provision of rehabilitation. Furthermore, they may offer additional mechanisms for promoting and tracking adherence to HEP. These tools may be utilised as an instrument to support existing rehabilitation processes and/or promote independent or remote rehabilitation. Amalgamating IoT-based technologies with gamification serves to promote creation of entertaining, customisable and accessible rehabilitation tools that suit a majority of individuals, irrespective of physical or cognitive capabilities [10].

Accordingly, this paper presents the preliminary findings of an exergame leveraging IoT. The Goalie exergame has been designed to support physiotherapeutic rehabilitation (within the clinic and remotely) for upper extremity pathologies. Modular development, applying the Design for Somebody (DfS) approach, was employed to support the use of the Goalie game by individuals with a range of capabilities.

2 Supporting Rehabilitation Adherence Through Technology

2.1 Leveraging IoT to Support HEP and Objective Data Collection

When quantifying adherence to HEP from a physiotherapeutic rehabilitation perspective, a number of factors are involved. These include how often the patient performs their HEP, the total amount of loading (quantity of the exercise, relating to time under tension and total number of repetitions performed) and whether this quantity is sufficient to provide a therapeutic benefit, and the duration the patient adheres to the HEP [11]. Unfortunately, it is challenging to accurately track adherence to HEP, as there appears to be a lack of reliable, validated measures to assess self-reported adherence [11]. For example, tools such as exercise diaries or logs require the patient to subjectively report completion of HEP. When utilising these reporting tools, 2.3 times higher dosage has been reported when compared to simultaneously recorded data from an electronic system [12]. Additionally, when compared to objective data measurements, as high as 90% of patients performed below the target exercise volume [12].

With the emergence of modern technologies such as IoT, it is becoming increasingly more economic to collect objective data measurements relating to HEP adherence [6]. IoT-based devices and sensor systems make it possible to capture detailed data about the quantity, quality and efficacy of rehabilitation programs. Accordingly, the possibility for widespread application of reliable and validated data collection tools reduces reliance on subjective, inherently inaccurate reporting systems. Incorporating these emerging technologies into HEP has the potential to remove subjectivity in reporting, thus supporting rehabilitation adherence and management by healthcare professionals.

2.2 *Rehabilitation Orientated Exergames*

Exergames can be identified as games providing encouragement to exercise, particularly for an audience that may be reluctant to engage in more traditional forms of exercise. Exergames are a commonly accepted method of encouraging physical activity, in an effort to promote health in individuals with high levels of sedentary behaviour [13]. The same exergaming ideology may also be applied within the healthcare and rehabilitation environment. To promote self-management strategies, the most successful new tools appear to incorporate two important factors: entertainment (self-motivation) and relevant therapeutic content (rehabilitation) [14].

Entertainment (relating to self-motivation) represents a challenge within rehabilitation and HEP. To date, factors negatively influencing HEP adherence are a multifactorial and poorly understood phenomenon [9]. Accordingly, this issue represents an impediment to effective rehabilitation, requiring additional investigation and the potential development of innovative modalities to enhance entertainment and adherence [9]. Exergaming represents one potential mechanism for promoting self-motivation through entertainment, in an effort to combat this challenge [8].

To ensure effective rehabilitation strategies, exergames should utilise relevant therapeutic content (with consideration towards the end-user's physical and cognitive capabilities). Currently, a majority of exergames are developed for the entertainment market, requiring a certain level of cognitive and physical capability for use. As such, many exergames fail to support gameplay for patients with impaired or compromised functionality, thus limiting their application within the rehabilitation environment [15]. This general-population focus may therefore not be appropriate to rehabilitation, as it fails to personalise gameplay for an individual's goals and performance level capabilities [8].

2.3 *Adapting Rehabilitation for Patients with Varying Capabilities*

The rehabilitation needs for patients can vary significantly. To ensure development of rehabilitation tools that suit a majority of individuals, irrespective of physical or cognitive capabilities, a "one-size fits all" strategy may not be appropriate. Novel strategies, such as the DfS approach, keep the end-user at the centre of the design process [16]. This facilitates creation of rehabilitation tools that can be customised for use by individuals with a range of capabilities [16].

A person, referring to an individual or very narrow target group, is at the centre of the DfS development process. DfS aims to serve target groups with highly specific needs, using a "bottom-up" philosophy (from small to all) [16]. To support this process, a modular design is key to individualised modification. Individual solutions (i.e., small) can then be adapted for wider user groups (i.e., all), through modifying these modules.

In the context of IoT-based rehabilitation exergames, a modular design with respect to gameplay settings facilitates adaption to suit individuals through to wider user groups. The ability to customise gameplay settings supports regression or progression of difficulty to suit the individual. As the individual advances through their rehabilitation, modifying gameplay settings supports progression, by adapting the level of challenge (difficulty and load) to the user's current performance level [8]. This principle may conversely be applied should performance drops. When considering physiotherapeutic exergames, these customisable gameplay settings need not be limited to physical functionality and may also support variations in cognition, visual and auditory capabilities.

3 Goalie Rehabilitation Exergame

The focus of this project was to develop an exergame, utilisable in musculoskeletal orientated rehabilitation by individuals with a wide range of capabilities. The Goalie game design was selected, as it provides a familiar construct within the Finnish environment (country of development), potentially reducing cognitive loading. To further reduce cognitive demand, gameplay was designed to mirror the user's movement pattern. Additionally, graphics were designed to be visually simple and intuitive.

The user interacts with the game using prescribed movement patterns (i.e., shoulder abduction). To monitor these movement patterns, the Goalie exergame utilises

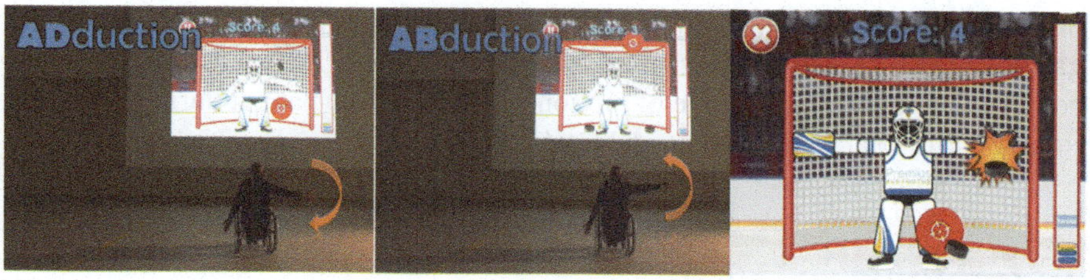

Fig. 1 Goalie exergame movement pattern and game image

specially manufactured sensors (controller) and a mobile device (display). These sensors are worn on the user's arms to track movement patterns, communicating with the exergame to mirror the physiotherapeutically prescribed exercise (i.e., movement pattern serves as a control input to the game) (Fig. 1).

Playing the game requires performance of shoulder abduction, raising the arms to prevent pucks entering the goal. Gameplay aims to promote muscular strength-endurance and improved range of motion around the shoulder. This movement was selected, as reduced upper extremity functionality is a common occurrence in many neurological conditions [17]. In addition, shoulder pain is a common musculoskeletal complaint, with prevalence ranging between 7 and 27% [18]. Shoulder pain and limitations in functionality can impact ability to perform basic activities of daily living (ADLs). This can subsequently result in loss of independence and inability to work, placing increased burden on the individual, family and the healthcare system.

Accordingly, shoulder abduction was selected as a rehabilitation exercise to promote strength and stability of the shoulder girdle, with a specific focus on the rotator cuff musculature. Shoulder abduction has demonstrated more balanced activation of rotator cuff musculature (supraspinatus, infraspinatus, subscapularis) when compared to shoulder flexion or extension movement patterns [19]. When performed in standing this movement pattern moves the whole shoulder girdle and so challenge not only the muscles of the cuff, but also the muscles of the scapula, trunk and arm. Additionally, this movement loads the rotator cuffs through increased ranges of movement. This increased range of motion can be beneficial to shoulder rehabilitation, as rotator cuffs are typically weakest just below shoulder height and above head height [19].

The game was designed using the DfS approach. In this game modularity is taken into account through a settings menu, in which the gameplay can be tailored for each individual and their rehabilitation needs. Variables including the patient's maximum range of motion, arms used for gameplay (left, right or both arms), number of repetitions, sets, speed of gameplay and recovery time may all be altered by the healthcare professional to facilitate exercise progression and use by individuals with a range of capabilities.

The associated gameplay data gathered from the sensors also facilitates tracking of HEP adherence, analysis of results by healthcare professionals and associated exercise progression. The necessary data was identified during the development process of the exergame, through consultation with healthcare professionals. Data gathered includes the number of repetitions performed for each arm, total sets completed, the maximum range of motion achieved by the patient during gameplay for each arm, total workout time and total rest time.

4 Conducting the Study

This initial prototype was designed to test the viability of such exergames within the rehabilitation environment, and whether they possess the potential to positively influence adherence. During the study, the game was played in a semi-controlled environment, with the rehabilitation professional facilitating game setup (attaching sensors to participants and defining gameplay settings specific to participant's rehabilitation requirements).

Participants for initial prototype testing ($N = 4$), included male (3) and female (1) patients within a rehabilitation centre. Participants ranged in age and encompassed a range of neurological conditions, including Parkinson's disease (PD), Amyotrophic lateral sclerosis (ALS) and paraplegia. The number of participants was intentionally kept rather small, since this study was supposed to be a preliminary trial focussing on qualitative findings (impact of exergame on motivation, suitability/complexity of exergame for varying patient groups, participant attitude to incorporating exergame into rehabilitation, etc.).

After playing, each participant was interviewed privately. A questionnaire was utilised to facilitate consistency in collation of participant's experience. The questionnaire consisted of questions relating to subjective experience about the exergame, general feel of the game, impact on motivation, complexity and comprehensibility of gameplay, usability of the equipment and ability of the exergame to support the participant's rehabilitation needs. In addition, the healthcare professionals ($N = 2$) responsible for testing's comments were collected to support this preliminary trial.

5 Results and Discussion

In general, the Goalie exergame received positive feedback. The game was seen to be a motivating, understandable and scalable tool for supporting the rehabilitation needs of patients. The main limitation in this trial was the relatively small test group, with a limited amount of data, which is why no conclusive findings can be made. However, initial results were promising, suggesting IoT-based rehabilitation exergames positively impact patient motivation and enjoyment.

Almost all patients participating in the trial found the scalability and associated gameplay difficulty to be suitable to their functional abilities. One participant found the game difficulty to be reasonably challenging. This patient possessed one of the more severe physical limitations in the test group, with PD typically impairing control and initiation of movement patterns. Notwithstanding, all patients agreed that the exergame supported their rehabilitation needs and would be interested in playing the game in the future. The participants stated that the Goalie exergame promoted self-motivation, serving to increase versatility in rehabilitation programming.

For the therapists (secondary user group), the game concept provided a new tool in rehabilitation, making it more versatile. When discussing the collected gameplay data, the therapists explained the game would be useful for remote rehabilitation, as a tool to motivate and monitor the progress of the client (and how/if the client is following their HEP). The ability to modify game parameters according to the needs and progress of the client was seen as extremely important. Allowing the therapist to adjust gameplay is lacking in most commercial exergames, which typically are not designed for rehabilitation or special user groups.

A significant factor that influences playability is related to the sensors' hardware. The sensors are attached to the patient's arm and connected to the exergame via Bluetooth. Participants found this initial setup to be slow. In addition, the sensors rely on single-axis rotation to determine arm position. As such, variations in arm or sensor position correlated with inaccuracy in the game's representation of arm position. Accordingly, participants identified the need for improvements to sensor hardware setup and robustness within gameplay.

Discussion with healthcare professionals responsible for testing also identified potential improvements to hardware. This included desired improvements to battery longevity and identification of an alternate use for the sensor technology. The participant's hardware concerns could be mitigated through adapted use of the sensors. The sensors may be attached to equipment typically utilised within rehabilitation (in particular, resistance machines). Attachment of sensors to resistance machines may also be beneficial to facilitating load progression. In addition, these resistance machines can be operated bilaterally or unilaterally, offering versatility for patients with varying capabilities. The resistance machines typically function in an arcing fashion, thus replicating the abduction movement pattern from the original gameplay. In addition to reducing set-up time, attaching the sensors to the resistance machine ensures sensors manoeuvre around a single-axis, resulting in increased accuracy.

Future development for the Goalie exergame involves improvement to the sensor hardware. As the sensor hardware capabilities develop, similarly the ability to monitor patient movement patterns and potential compensations improves. In addition, the Goalie exergame developed under this project is relatively simple. As such, gameplay may provide limited entertainment over extended periods of use. Another future development involves additional mini-exergames, incorporating elements commonly associated with gamified applications to enhance motivation. Future iterations of the game shall also allow modification of audio and graphics to suit the user's sensory (visual and auditory) requirements and interests. This was considered during game design, although in this early version only one graphics setting was utilised.

6 Conclusions

This study demonstrated encouraging results regarding the utilisation of IoT-based exergames in rehabilitation to increase adherence to HEP. Utilisation of exergames in the rehabilitation setting is considered a viable tool for providing entertaining (self-motivating) rehabilitation. Exergames combined with IoT technologies also facilitate development of customisable rehabilitation tools which allow gameplay setting customisation to suit a majority of individuals, irrespective of physical or cognitive capabilities. In this study, the Goalie exergame was introduced and authentic user experiences related to the usability and suitability were investigated. Both therapists and patients were included in the study. The application of the game to rehabilitation was considered moderately feasible with respect to usability, but there is need for further improvements. In particular, the IoT technology utilised requires further refinement. Additional functions to further promote gameplay and self-motivation should also be integrated in the future.

References

1. Official Statistics of Finland: Population structure [e-publication]. Statistics Finland, Helsinki. ISSN=1797–5395. http://www.stat.fi/til/vaerak/index_en.html (2017). Accessed 17 Jan 2018
2. McNicoll, G.: World population ageing 1950-2050. Popul. Dev. Rev. **28**(4), 814–816 (2002)
3. Denton, F.T., Spencer, B.G.: Chronic health conditions: changing prevalence in an aging population and some implications for the delivery of health care services. Can. J. Aging. **29**(1), 11–21 (2010)
4. Gubbi, J., Buyya, R., Marusic, S., Palaniswami, M.: Internet of things (IoT): a vision, architectural elements, and future directions. Futur. Gener. Comput. Syst. **29**(7), 1645–1660 (2013)
5. Yan, L., Zhang, Y., Yang, L.T., Ning, H. (eds.): The Internet of Things: from RFID to the Next-Generation Pervasive Networked Systems. CRC Press, Boca Raton (2008)
6. Almotiri, S.H., Khan, M.A., Alghamdi, M.A.: Mobile health (m-health) system in the context of IoT. In: Future Internet of Things and Cloud Workshops (FiCloudW), IEEE International Conference on, pp. 39–42. IEEE (2016)
7. Philip, V., Suman, V.K., Menon, V.G., Dhanya, K.A.: A review on latest internet of things based healthcare applications. Int. J. Comput. Sci. Inf. Secur. **15**(1), 248 (2017)
8. Skjæret, N., Nawaz, A., Morat, T., Schoene, D., Helbostad, J.L., Vereijken, B.: Exercise and rehabilitation delivered through exergames in older adults: an integrative review of technologies, safety and efficacy. Int. J. Med. Inform. **85**(1), 1–16 (2016)
9. Rizzo, J.: Patients' mental models and adherence to outpatient physical therapy home exercise programs. Physiother. Theory Pract. **31**(4), 253–259 (2015)
10. Klasnja, P., Pratt, W.: Healthcare in the pocket: mapping the space of mobile-phone health interventions. J. Biomed. Inform. **45**(1), 184–198 (2012)
11. Bollen, J.C., Dean, S.G., Siegert, R.J., Howe, T.E., Goodwin, V.A.: A systematic review of measures of self-reported adherence to unsupervised home-based rehabilitation exercise programmes, and their psychometric properties. BMJ Open. **4**(6), e005044 (2014)
12. Rathleff, M.S., Bandholm, T., McGirr, K.A., Harring, S.I., Sørensen, A.S., Thorborg, K.: New exercise-integrated technology can monitor the dosage and quality of exercise performed against an elastic resistance band by adolescents with patellofemoral pain: an observational study. J. Physiother. **62**(3), 159–163 (2016)

13. Whitehead, A., Johnston, H., Nixon, N., Welch, J.: Exergame effectiveness: what the numbers can tell us. In: Proceedings of the 5th ACM SIGGRAPH Symposium on Video Games, pp. 55–62. ACM, New York (2010)
14. Merilampi, S., Koivisto, A., Sirkka, A., Raumonen, P., Virkki, J., Xiao, X., et al.: The cognitive mobile games for older adults - a Chinese user experience study. In: Serious Games and Applications for Health (SeGAH), 2017 IEEE 5th International Conference on, pp. 1–6. IEEE (2017)
15. Wüest, S., Langenberg, R., Bruin, E.D.: Design considerations for a theory-driven exergame-based rehabilitation program to improve walking of persons with stroke. Eur. Rev. Aging Phys. Act. **11**(2), 119 (2014)
16. Sirkka, A., Merilampi, S., Koivisto, A., Tommiska, J., Saarinen, T.-P.: "Design for Somebody" - approach enabling mobile technology development. Stud. Health Technol. Inform. **242**, 669–675 (2017)
17. Carroll, D.: A quantitative test of upper extremity function. J. Chronic Dis. **18**(5), 479–491 (1965)
18. Luime, J.J., Koes, B.W., Hendriksen, I.J.M., Burdorf, A., Verhagen, A.P., Miedema, H.S., Verhaar, J.A.N.: Prevalence and incidence of shoulder pain in the general population; a systematic review. Scand. J. Rheumatol. **33**(2), 73–81 (2004)
19. Wattanaprakornkul, D., Cathers, I., Halaki, M., Ginn, K.A.: The rotator cuff muscles have a direction specific recruitment pattern during shoulder flexion and extension exercises. J. Sci. Med. Sport. **14**(5), 376–382 (2011)

Context Awareness as Resource for Monitoring Elderly Depressed

Edwing Almeida Calderón, Marcela Buitrón de la Torre, and Marco Ferruzca Navarro

1 Extended Abstract: The Context Awareness as Resource for Monitoring Elderly Depressed People

1.1 Context Awareness and Disruptive Technology

This case study was made since the Industrial Design Approach, working interdisciplinary with Psychologist and Geriatrics.

The concept of context awareness (CA) arises from ubiquitous computing [1] and its objective is to acquire and use information that allows identifying the situation in which an entity is located [2], whether an object, a person, or both.

The Internet of Things (IoT) allows us to interconnect different devices capable of sensing environmental, physical environmental situations such as temperature, illumination, movement, sound, etc. [3]. The CA gives escalation to multiple proposals to improve the quality of life of users. One, specifically, is e-health or telemedicine. This concept visualizes distance medical consultation, medical treatment, or monitoring of different patients with different types of diseases or conditions.

The disruptive systems [4] and open hardware like microcontrollers such as the Arduino, Raspberry Pi, Onion, Intel Galileo, among others, coupled with the emergence of various sensors allow to identify situations that occur in the day-to-day of people.

E. Almeida Calderón (✉) · M. Buitrón de la Torre · M. Ferruzca Navarro
Universidad Autónoma Metropolitana, Ciudad de México, Mexico
e-mail: eaac@correo.azc.uam.mx; meb@correo.azc.uam.mx; mvfn@correo.azc.uam.mx

P. R. M. Inácio et al. (eds.), *5th EAI International Conference on IoT Technologies for HealthCare*, EAI/Springer Innovations in Communication and Computing,
https://doi.org/10.1007/978-3-030-30335-8_10

1.2 Monitoring Elderly Depressed

Several countries are experiencing a process of aging of their population, where the world population is expected to exceed nine billion people by 2050 [5], two billion more than at present. The increase will take place almost entirely in developing countries. In Mexico, an increase of 3–5% for the year 2050 of the population over 85 years old [6].

In Mexico, the INEGI[1] considers older people the population of 60 years or older [7], the current situation and the perception of society, has forced to establish different ranges for the older adults, setting tree levels of older adults: young older adult (65 and 75 years old), older adult (75 and 85 years old) and older advanced adult (+85 years old) [8]. Last ones present a high or total loss of autonomy, more prone to vulnerability and generate greater demands in terms of attention and resources [5]. This condition of disability is reflected in the change in activities of daily living (Activity of Daily Living, ADL) [9], people report one or more severe limitations, defined as a central set of care activities or personal self-care [6], directly affecting the family, since as the disability increases, care work will be assumed and in many cases the State will have to assume treatments, medicines, and even the care [8].

Depression is one of the most common psychiatric conditions in older adults; however, continuously this condition is poorly diagnosed and poorly treated [10]. This leads to many consequences such as the increase in the cost of patient treatment and family problems [11]. It conditions increases cost to society [12], represented by millions in the payment of treatments, medicines, hospitalization, and goes directly to the treasury, to relatives and in some cases the patients lack resources to be able to carry out a treatment [13].

The diagnosis of depression is determined by the application of a questionnaire. In Mexico, the instrument designed by the ENASEM (National Study on Health and Aging in Mexico) is applied, which ensures a reliability of 80.7% [9]. The correct diagnosis gets more difficult when the ailments are accompanied by chronic diseases. The factor of ADL, conditions of loneliness coupled with the symptoms may be masked by other conditions, including the conditions of the natural deterioration of aging [14].

There is no physiological or biological analysis such as a blood test or similar to confirm a diagnosis of depression [15]. Some studies to determine the relationship of biological–physiological markers that help determine a state of depression. Suraki [16] proposes a methodology to make a diagnosis, based on the ADL. However, they do not correlate physiological data or biomarkers for this diagnosis and do not give proof of the reliability of the method.

The case study is presented for the monitoring of elderly people in a depressed state with the objective of assessing the utility and perceived contribution. The sys-

[1]INEGI: (NIIG, National Institute of Information and Statistics in Mexico).

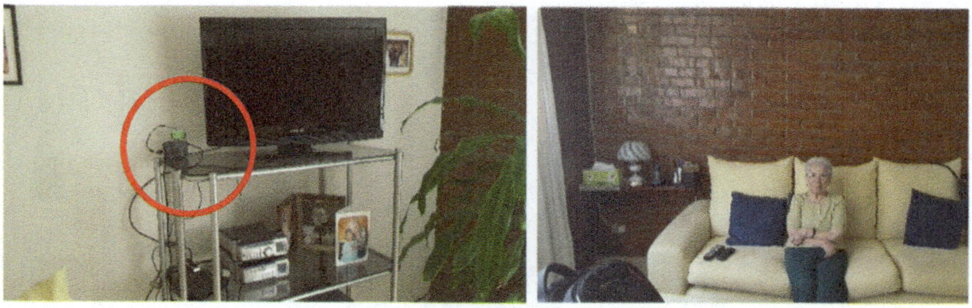

Image 1 Placement of the system for the best visualization of the ADL

tem was tested (initially) with three patients, under the medical protocol established for this purpose, seeking to identify the operation, advantages or disadvantages, and the knowledge of the patient's user experience, the family member, and the treating physician. In other words, the U/X user experience will be evaluated.

The system was applied to "healthy" elderly patients aged +70 years previously diagnosed of depressive state. The patient must wear a bracelet (left arm preferred) and will be monitored in his ADL. Secondary user: family caregiver must install the system (place, connect, put the bracelet), charge and change batteries, check operation on the website. The medical user: not physical contact, monitorize through the website (http://www.cixxi.com.mx/finch/index.php).

The use of the bracelet was for 24 h a day and 2 weeks for a minimum period. In the first week, the system registers and learns the patient's ADL. In the second week, the system has "learned" the ADL and begins the comparison with respect to the record of the previous week, by day and time.

Figure 1 shows the configuration of the system. At first point is a bracelet that acquires biomarkers such as temperature and hear rate. Its information is sent to a second module constructed in a Raspberry Pi configured with Open CV for recognition of human body and track person movement to register the ADL. That information is collected into a server and it presents the information in a Website to the family or caregiver and the medic responsive, via Internet.

The results of the system application are displayed on the website for each patient. Identifying the patient's image, data or observations to it, the temperature and heart rate by date and time, as well as the ADL map with a background image. The system sends a series of alerts by SMS or email, also at the when the system starts.

The system identifies human bodies and records their position at each moment in Cartesian coordinates within a plane, this plane is the image captured by the camera.

Figure 2 presents an example. Superimposed on the background image, the tracking map. The places of incidence of the patient, where the dark pictures (blue) indicate little presence or movement. The yellow boxes indicate the greatest amount of incidence or movement. A grid that facilitates the location of the Cartesian map area.

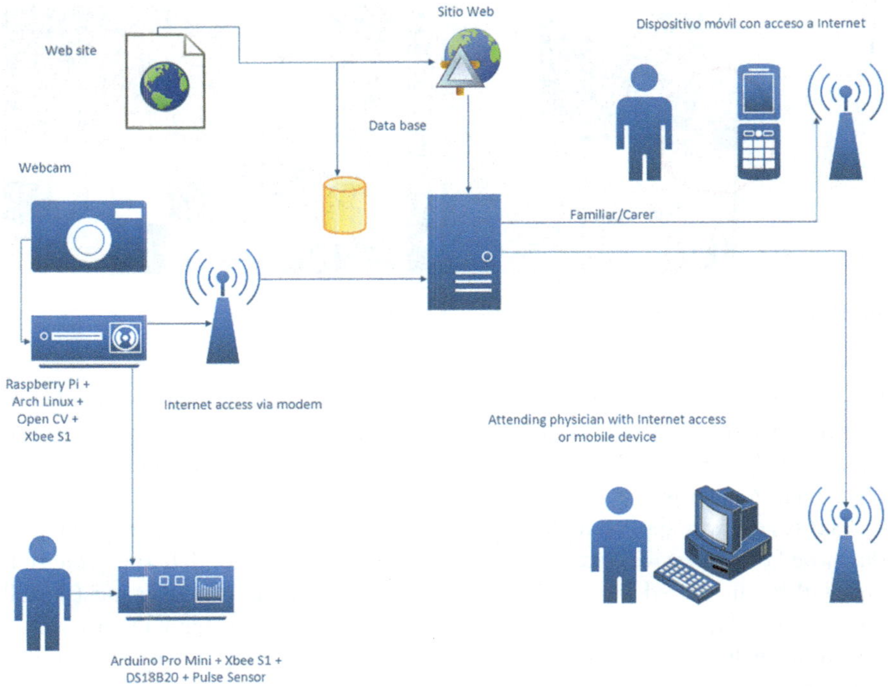

Fig. 1 System proposal, configuration, and system function

User Experience from Patients (U/X)

Once the monitoring process was completed, the survey was applied to the patient, the family member or caregiver, and the doctor or treating person. The intention of this interrogation was to know the UX of the users. It seeks to identify the acceptance of the use of technology for monitoring in older adults.

The responses of the patients allowed us to identify the level of acceptance of the system and the ergonomic appearance of the bracelet and the ease of use of it. Patients willingly accepted the application of this and showed no fear or any doubt about the use of it. There was unanimity in the system's parentage and everyone reports benefit when applying the monitoring in their ADL. In general, it is thought that it is a good idea and that it can help them in their well-being.

In the same way, the idea that the patient warns family members in case of an emergency or readings that are in the alert range (high temperature, HR, or alterations in the ADL) was good. What is interesting is knowing that everyone prefers to be notified to family members and not to the doctor or trader.

The relatives of the patients accepted the proposal well. Seeing that the system is not invasive and there is no need to install special facilities and it can be placed practically anywhere in the house, it improves the acceptance of it and normally

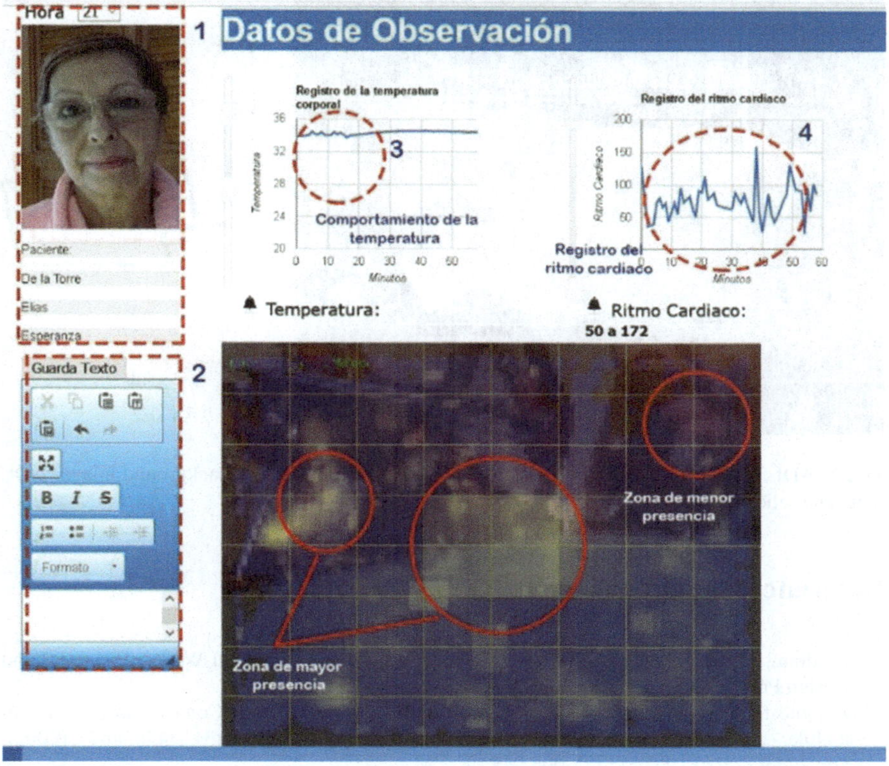

Image 2 View of the website for the doctor or family member. (1) Photograph of the patient; (2) Space to add annotations; (3) Temperature graph per hour; (4) HR chart per hour; (5) Map of ADL

they do not even notice the presence of it, until you tell them where it was placed and how.

The acceptance of the placement and monitoring of their relatives was also as expected. Since, although there was some doubt at the beginning, when seeing that they did not require special knowledge or to be attentive to the functioning of the system, the family members expressed greater taste and acceptance of the proposal.

Regarding security, when seeing the results of the images taken from the ADL, the relatives refer to it as they clearly see that there is no invasion of their privacy and the results can be interpreted, even by them. Relatives.

There is an area of opportunity and that is the duration, recharge, and change of the battery. This is due to the duration of only 12 h, to the “difficulty” of placement and even the visualization of the operation of the bracelet.

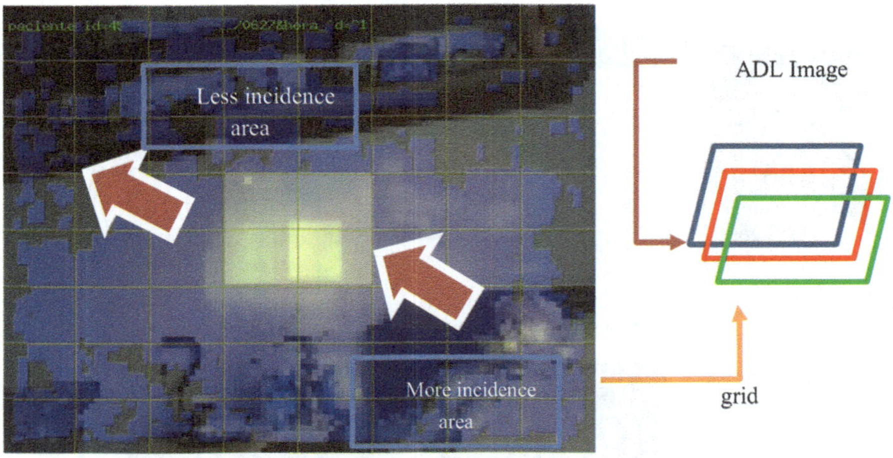

Fig. 2 ADL capture resulting in Cartesian image map in three layers: Background image, ADL map, and reticle

References

1. Bardram, J.E.: Applications of Context-Aware Computing in Hospital Work – Examples and Design Principles. ACM, New York (2004)
2. Anagnostopoulos, C.B., Tsounis, A., Hadjiefthymiades, S.: Context awareness in mobile computing environments. Wirel. Pers. Commun. **42**(3), 445–464 (2006). https://doi.org/10.1007/s11277-006-9187-6
3. Choi, W., Kim, S., Keum, M., Han, D.K., Ko, H., Member, S.: Acoustic and visual signal based context awareness system for mobile application. IEEE Trans. Consum. Electron. **57**(2), 738–746 (2011)
4. Sundmaeker, H., Saint-exupéry, A.D.: Vision and challenges for realising the internet of things. Clust. Eur. Res. Proj. Internet Things Eur. Comm. **3**(3), 34–36 (2010)
5. OECD: Science and technology perspectives on an ageing society. In: OECD Science, Technology and Industry Outlook 2012. OECD, Paris (2012). https://doi.org/10.1787/sti_outlook-2012-en
6. Lafortune, G., Balestat, G.: OECD health working papers no. 26. In: Trends in Severe Disability Among Elderly People, p. 81. OECD, Paris (2007). https://doi.org/10.1787/217072070078
7. INEGI: Los Adultos Mayores en México. Perfil sociodemográfico al Inicio del Siglo XXI, 2005th edn. INEGI, Aguascalientes (2005)
8. Haberkern, K., Schmid, T., Neuberger, F., Grignon, M.: The role of the elderly as providers and recipients of care. In: The Future of Families to 2030. OECD, Paris (2011). https://doi.org/10.1787/9789264168367-en
9. Yáñez-luis, M.M.C.J.A., Fernández-Guzmán, C.M.C.M.P., De Brigada, G., Manuel, M.C.V.: Características clinimétricas en adultos mayores consultados en la. Especialidad de Geriatría de la Unidad de Especialidades Médicas. **63**(4), 156–177 (2009)
10. Crawford, M.J., Prince, M., Menezes, P., Mann, H.: The recognition and treatment of depression in older people. Int. J. Og Geriatr. Psychiatr. **13**(December 1997), 172176 (1998)
11. Cullum, S., Tucker, S., Todd, C., Brayne, C.: Screening for depression in older medical inpatients. Int. J. Geriatr. Psychiatry. **21**(5), 469–476 (2006). https://doi.org/10.1002/gps.1497
12. Mavis, E.: Detection and management of depression in the elderly physically I11 patient. Human Psycopharmacol. **10**, 235–241 (1995). http://doi.org/0885-6222/95/S40235-07

13. Bonin-guillaume, S., Sautel, L., Demattei, C., Jouve, E., Blin, O.: Validation of the retardation rating scale for detecting depression in geriatric inpatients. Int. J. Geriatr. Psychiatry. **22**(1), 68–76 (2007). https://doi.org/10.1002/gps.1657
14. Dorfman, R.A., Lubben, J.E., Mayer-Oakes, A., Atchison, K., Schweitzer, S.O., De Jong, F.J., Matthias, R.E.: Screening for depression among a well elderly population. Soc. Work. **40**(3), 295–304 (1995)
15. Albrecht, A.M., Herrick, C.M.: 100 preguntas y respuestas sobre la depresión, 2nd edn. EDAF, Madrid (2007)
16. Suraki, M.Y., Suraki, M.Y., Nejati, O.: Benefit of internet of things to improve business interaction with depression prevention and treatment. In: 2012 IEEE 14th International Conference on E-Health Networking, Applications and Services (Healthcom), pp. 403–406. IEEE (2012). https://doi.org/10.1109/HealthCom.2012.6379448

Index

P. R. M. Inácio et al. (eds.), *5th EAI International Conference on IoT Technologies for HealthCare*, EAI/Springer Innovations in Communication and Computing,
https://doi.org/10.1007/978-3-030-30335-8

The manufacturer's authorised representative in the EU is Springer Nature Customer Service Centre GmbH, Europaplatz 3, 69115 Heidelberg, Germany. If you have any concerns regarding our products, please contact ProductSafety@springernature.com

Printed and bound by CPI Group (UK) Ltd, Croydon, CR0 4YY

30/09/2026

02225259-0003